W9-BYH-494

USMLE STEP 1 RECALL
Buzzwords for the Boards
Second Edition

RECALL SERIES EDITOR

LORNE H. BLACKBOURNE, M.D.
Fellow, Trauma/Critical Care
Department of Surgery
University of Miami
Jackson Memorial Hospital
Miami, Florida

USMLE STEP 1 RECALL
Buzzwords for the Boards
Second Edition

BRENT A. REINHEIMER, M.D.
Hospitalist/House Doctor
Community Medical Center
An affiliation of St. Barnabas Health Care System
Toms River, New Jersey

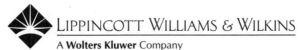

LIPPINCOTT WILLIAMS & WILKINS
A **Wolters Kluwer** Company
Philadelphia · Baltimore · New York · London
Buenos Aires · Hong Kong · Sydney · Tokyo

Senior Acquisitions Editor: Neil Marquardt
Development Editor: Beth Goldner
Senior Marketing Manager: Scott Lavine
Project Editor: Caroline Define
Designer: Doug Smock
Typesetter: Peirce Graphic Services
Printer: R.R. Donnelley & Sons

351 West Camden Street
Baltimore, Maryland 21201-2436 USA

530 Walnut Street
Philadelphia, Pennsylvania 19106

Printed in the United States of America

Library of Congress Cataloging-in-Publication Data

Reinheimer, Brent A.
    USMLE step 1 recall : buzzwords for the boards / Brent A. Reinheimer. — 2nd ed.
        p. cm.
    Includes bibliographical references and index.
    ISBN 0-7817-4513-6
    1. Medical sciences — Examinations, questions, etc. 2. Medical sciences —
Outlines, syllabi, etc. I. Title: USMLE step one recall. II. Title.

R834.5.R44 2004
610'.76—dc22   2003066027

The publishers have made every effort to trace the copyright holders for borrowed material. If they have inadvertently overlooked any, they will be pleased to make the necessary arrangements at the first opportunity.

05 06 07 08 09
1 2 3 4 5 6 7 8 9 1

Preface

ABOUT THE BOARDS

Step I is designed to see whether a student can understand and apply the basic sciences to the practice of medicine. The exam is written in a multiple choice format. A majority of the questions will include graphs or tables that you will need to interpret. Still other questions may require you to identify gross or microscopic specimens, both normal and pathologic.

What was once traditionally divided into anatomy, behavioral science, biochemistry, microbiology, immunology, physiology, pharmacology, and pathology sections are now categorized differently. The content hasn't changed (albeit expanded), but the names we call them have. Regarding Step I, the basic sciences are broken down according to whether the questions focus on concepts and principles that are germane to an organ system or to organ *systems*. From this point, they can be further subdivided on a myriad of things; environmental, psychosocial, normal, abnormal, therapy, and the like.

I am still no better on a computer than I was while writing the first edition of this manual, and yet I was able to navigate through the website *www.usmle.org/ step1* with ease. It is self-explanatory and will provide you with all the answers to your questions regarding Step I. Content description, the application process, test-taking sites, and tutorials can all be found there.

Applying for the USMLE Step I depends on whether you are a student or graduate of a United States accredited Medical school or are outside the US and Canada. US and Canadian accredited medical students need to contact the NBME. Their contact information is Examinee Support Services, 3750 Market Street, Philadelphia, PA 19104-3190; website: *http://www.nbme.org;* telephone (215) 590–9700. Foreign medical students and graduates need to contact the ECFMG at 3624 Market Street, Philadelphia, PA 19104-2685; website: *http://www.ecfmg.org;* telephone (215) 386-5900.

You will receive a packet of information regarding your USMLE Step I application. It will contain your scheduling permit and instructions on how to contact Prometric to schedule your exam. I suggest using the website: *http://www. prometric.com* for current locations and times available for test taking.

ABOUT THE BOOK

USMLE Step I Recall: Buzzwords for the Boards, second edition, evolved from my study notes for the Step I exam. As I studied a particular topic, I took the "high yield" facts and arranged them into questions that I placed on the left side of the page, with the corresponding correct answers on the right (same format you will see throughout this book). The questions were written in such a manner that the answer could be short, which allowed me to review large volumes of information in a relatively short period of time. What I used to do was take a blank sheet of paper, fold it lengthwise and cover the answers in the right hand column. A bookmark is provided for you to do the same.

I often studied with friends, and soon they began to ask me for copies of my "buzzwords" (so named because they were composed of high yield facts). In exchange for my notes, my only request to my friends was that they proofread the questions and answers. After using "buzzwords," my friends began insisting that it should be published. As more people told me to publish the material, I began to consider reworking the material for publication.

After taking the Step I exam, I realized how well my "buzzwords" had helped me answer the questions. At that point, I continued to work on the manual, refining, adding, deleting, and correcting questions for the next 18 months. It soon became apparent that the question and answer nature of my original study guide enabled it to fit well into the Lippincott Williams & Wilkins *Recall* series of books. *USMLE Step I Recall: Buzzwords for the Boards,* first edition, was published in 1999.

In October 2001, I decided it was time for an update. Several things needed to occur for this to be accomplished. The nature of the book's format makes review of the material nearly impossible because the questions are randomized within each chapter. What I decided was to re-write the entire manual, but while doing this, I would arrange questions into "q-banks" (an example would be Physiology/Pulmonary). Also, back at LWW, they would begin breaking the original manual into the respective question banks that I provided for them. We then merged the two "q-banks" of questions from the first manual and my new re-write, chose a predetermined number of questions from their respective banks, and randomized them into the book you see here today.

Each student has their own particular strengths and weaknesses and, therefore, will assign their own importance to a particular chapter. It is completely individual. Therefore, the chapter order of *USMLE Step I Recall: Buzzwords for the Boards,* second edition, is arranged in what I consider the most logical progression instead of "importance." The anatomical chapter is placed first, because I believe the four subtopics (Embryology, Histology, Neuroscience, and Gross Anatomy) are the foundations of medical knowledge. I placed the Behavioral Science chapter next to increase the likelihood of it being seen and read more frequently than if it was placed at the end of the book, because it is the section students historically leave for last, and therefore is the least reviewed (I know this from a first hand experience). The Pathology chapter is the last (before the Power Review) because it encompasses all other aspects of the basic sciences, from general to cellular to physiological. Students need to have a complete understanding of "normal" body function before they can fully comprehend how a disease can affect function.

The "Power Review" chapter of the book is a compilation of helpful hints I have amassed in preparing for the medical boards. These "buzzwords" should be an enormous help to you while taking Step I; they act like "neon signs" advertising the answer. Buzzwords, Most Commons, Chromosomes, Vitamins and Minerals, and Antidotes were taken out of their respective chapters with the hope of drawing your attention to them and, therefore, increasing the likelihood of you answering them correctly on the exam. A formula and equation appendix was also added to this edition. The appendix does not include every equation known, but it does include the "major players" and should be of great service to you. My feeling was that they could become "lost in the shuffle" if they had not been placed into their own section.

An interesting aspect of the Step I exam is the random nature of the questions; they are not grouped by subject matter. The purpose of this approach is to test your complete knowledge on any and all basic sciences rather than one particular topic. For this reason, the questions within each chapter of *USMLE Step I Recall: Buzzwords for the Boards* are presented "at random"—that is, for the most part, they are not grouped together by subtopics within the main chapter. This will help you prepare for the random presentation of the questions found in the USMLE Step I exam, albeit on a far lesser scale.

Once you feel you have mastered a particular subject area, use the related chapter in this book to test your actual level of knowledge. When studying with a friend or friends, pick a chapter and question each other. When you ask a question, not only are you questioning your study partner, but if you cover the answer with the bookmark provided, you too need to come up with the correct answer.

SUMMARY

The structure of this study guide emphasizes the reinforcement rather than the attainment of knowledge. This manual is not intended to be used on a one-time basis. Rather, you should review the book as many times as necessary to successfully answer all of the questions. There really is no right or wrong way to use this book (barring not using it at all). However, you should use it in the manner that will allow you to pass "The Boards."

USMLE Step I Recall: Buzzwords for the Boards is NOT intended to replace your conventional textbooks, but rather to supplement your textbooks and class/lecture notes. If used in conjunction with your primary texts, this study guide will be extremely beneficial in helping you achieve a successful result in the USMLE Step I examination. By faithfully reviewing your texts, notes, and this study guide, you will increase your chances of passing this most challenging of exams. Good luck on the test and just remember: repetition is the cornerstone of learning medicine.

Contents

Common Abbreviations

AA	amino acid
AADC	amino acid decarboxylase
Ab(s)	antibody (ies)
ACE	angiotensin converting enzyme
ACh	acetylcholine
ACL	anterior cruciate ligament
ACTH	adrenocorticotrophic hormone
AD	autosomal dominant
ADCC	antibody-dependent cell-mediated cytotoxicity
ADH	antidiuretic hormone
ADHD	attention deficit hyperactive disorder
ADP	adenosine diphosphate
Ag	antigen
AICA	anterior inferior cerebellar artery
AIDS	acquired immunodeficiency syndrome
ALA	aminolevulinic acid
ALL	acute lymphocytic leukemia, also called acute lymphoblastic anemia
AlPO$_4$	aluminum phosphate
AML	acute myelocytic leukemia
AMP	adenosine monophosphate
ANA	antinuclear antibody
ANOVA	analysis of variance
ANS	autonomic nervous system
APC	antigen-presenting cell
apo	apolipoprotein
AR	autosomal recessive
ASA	acetylsalicylic acid (aspirin)
ASD	atrial septal defect
ASO	antistreptolysin O
AT II	angiotensin II
AT III	angiotensin III
ATP	adenosine 5' triphosphate
ATPase	adenine triphosphatase

AV	arteriovenous or atrioventricular
AZT	azidothymidine
BP	blood pressure
2,3-BPG	2,3-bisphosphoglycerate
BPH	benign prostatic hyperplasia
CA	cancer antigen
cAMP	cyclic adenosine monophosphate
C-ANCA	cytoplasmic antineutrophilic cytoplasmic antibody
CAP	catabolite activation protein
CCK	cholecystokinin
CDC	Centers for Disease Control and Prevention
cDNA	copy deoxyribonucleic acid
CEA	carcinoembryonic antigen
CGD	chronic granulomatous disease
CHF	congestive heart failure
CHO	carbohydrate
CLL	chronic lymphocytic leukemia
CML	chronic myelocytic leukemia
CMV	cytomegalovirus
CN	cranial nerve
CNS	central nervous system
CO	carbon monoxide
CoA	coenzyme A
COMT	catechol-*O*-methyl transferase
Cox-2	cyclooxygenase 2
CPK	creatinine phosphokinase
CPR	cardiopulmonary resuscitation
CREST syndrome	a variant of scleroderma characterized by *c*alcinosis, *R*aynaud's phenomenon, *e*sophageal motility disorders, *s*clerodactyly, and *t*elangiectasia
CRH	cortisol-releasing hormone
CSF	cerebrospinal fluid
DAG	diacylglycerol
DCML	dorsal column-medial lemniscus
DCT	distal collecting tubule
DHEA	dehydroepiandrosterone
DIC	disseminated intravascular coagulation
DIP	distal interphalangeal (joint)
DLCO	carbon monxide diffusion in the lung
DM	diabetes mellitus
DNA	deoxyribonucleic acid
DOC	drug of choice
ds	double stranded

DSM-IV	Diagnostic and Statistical Manual of Mental Disorders - Fourth Edition
DVT	deep vein thrombosis
EBV	Epstein-Barr virus
ECF	extracellular fluid
ECG	electrocardiogram
ED_{50}	median effective dose
EDV	end-diastolic volume
EDTA	ethylenediaminetetraacetic acid
EEG	electroencephalogram
eEF	elongation factor
eIF	initiation factor
ELISA	enzyme-linked immunosorbent assay
EPS	extrapyramidal syndrome
EPSP	excitatory postsynaptic potential
ER	emergency room
ERPF	effective renal plasma flow
ERV	expiratory reserve volume
ESR	erythrocyte sedimentation rate
ESV	end-systolic volume
ETC	electron transport chain
F	female
Fab	fragment, antigen-binding
$FADH_2$	reduced form of flavin adenine dinucleotide
FDA	US Food and Drug Administration
FEV	forced expiratory volume
FEV_1	forced expiratory volume in 1 second
FF	filtration fraction
FiO_2	fractional concentration of oxygen in inspired gas
fL	femtoliters
FRC	functional residual capacity
FSH	follicle-stimulating hormone
5-FU	5-fluorouracil
GABA	gamma-aminobutyric acid
GBM	glomerular basement membrane
GDPH	glycerol-3-phosphate dehydrogenase
GERD	gastroesophageal reflux disease
GFAP	glial fibrillary acidic protein
GFR	glomerular filtration rate
GH	growth hormone
GHRH	growth hormone-releasing hormone
GI	gastrointestinal
GLUT	glucose transporter

GMP	guanylic acid
GN	glomerular nephritis (glomerulonephritis)
GnRH	gonadotropin-releasing hormone
GP	glycoprotein
GP41	glycoprotein 41
G-6-PD	glucose-6-phosphate dehydrogenase
GTP	guanosine triphosphate
HAV	hepatitis A virus
HB$_c$Ab/Ag	hepatitis C antibody/antigen
HB$_e$Ab/Ag	hepatitis E antibody/antigen
HB$_s$Ab/Ag	hepatitis B surface antibody/antigen
HBV	hepatitis B virus
Hgb	hemoglobin
hCG	human chorionic gonadotropin
HCl	hydrochloric acid
HCO$_3{}^-$	bicarbonate
hCS	human chorionic somatomammotropin
Hct	hematocrit
HDL	high-density lipoprotein
HGPRT	hypoxanthine guanine phosphoribosyl transferase
HHV	human herpesvirus
5-HIAA	5-hydroxyindoleacetic acid
HIV	human immunodeficiency virus
HLA	human leukocyte antigen
HMG-CoA	3-hydroxy-3-methyl-glutaryl coenzyme A
HMP	hexose monophosphate
hnRNA	heterogenous nuclear ribonucleic acid
H$_2$O	water
H$_2$O$_2$	hydrogen peroxide
HPV	human papilloma virus
HSV	herpes simplex virus
5-HT	5-hydroxytryptamine (serotonin)
HTLV	human T-cell leukemia virus
HTN	hypertension
ICF	intracellular fluid
IDL	intermediate-density lipoprotein
IF	intrinsic factor
IFN-α	interferon-α
Ig	immunoglobulin
IGF-1	insulin-like growth factor type 1
IL	interleukin
IM	intramuscular
IMP	inosine 5′-monophosphate (inosinic acid)

IP$_3$	inositol triphosphate
IQ	intelligent quotient
IRV	inspiratory reserve volume
ITP	idiopathic thrombocytopenia
IV	intravenous/intravenously
IVC	inferior vena cava
JG	juxtaglomerular
KOH	potassium hydroxide
L	liter
LAP	leukocyte alkaline phosphatase
LD$_{50}$	median lethal dose
LDH	lactate dehydrogenase
LDL	low-density lipoprotein
LGB	lateral geniculate body
LH	luteinizing hormone
LMN	lower motor neuron
LT	leukotriene
M	male
MAC	membrane attack complex
MAO	monoamine oxidase
MAOI	monoamine oxidase inhibitor
MCC	most common cause
MCH	mean corpuscular hemoglobin
MCHC	mean corpuscular hemoglobin concentration
MCV	mean corpuscular volume
MEN	multiple endocrine neoplasia
MGB	medial geniculate body
MGN	membranous glomerulonephritis
MHC	major histocompatibility complex
MI	myocardial infarction
MIF	müllerian inhibiting factor
MPGN	membranoproliferative glomerulonephritis
mRNA	messenger ribonucleic acid
MRSA	methicillin-resistant *Staphylococcus aureus*
NaCl	sodium chloride (table salt)
NADH	reduced nicotinamide adenine dinucleotide
NADPH	reduced nicotinamide adenine dinucleotide phosphate
NE	norepinephrine
NK cells	natural killer cells
NMJ	neuromuscular junction
NO	nitric oxide
NPH	normal pressure hydrocephalus
NREM	nonrapid eye movement

NRDS	neonatal respiratory distress syndrome
NSAID	nonsteroidal anti-inflammatory drug
OAA	oxaloacetate
OCD	obsessive-compulsive disorder
OCP	oral contraceptive pill
$-OH$	hydroxy
p50	oxygen tension at 50% saturation of blood
$PaCO_2$	arterial carbon dioxide pressure
PAH	para-aminohippurate
PALS	parietolateral lymphocyte sheath
PAM	pralidoxime
P-ANCA	perinuclear anti-neutrophilic cytoplasmic antibody
PaO_2	arterial oxygen pressure
PAS	periodic acid-Schiff (test)
P_{CO2}	partial pressure of carbon dioxide
PCR	polymerase chain reaction
PCT	proximal convoluted tubule
PDA	patent ductus arteriosus
PDE	phosphodiester
PEPCK	phosphoenolpyruvate carboxykinase
PFK-1	phosphofructokinase-1
PG	prostaglandin
pI	isoelectric point
PICA	posterior inferior cerebellar artery
PIF	prolactin-inhibiting factor
PIP	proximal interphalangeal (joint)
PKU	phenylketonuria
PMN	polymorphonucleocyte
PNMT	phenylethanolamine N-methyltransferase
PNS	peripheral nervous system
P_{O2}	partial pressure of oxygen
$PO_4{}^-$	phosphate
POMC	pro-opiomelanocortin
PPD test	purified protein derivative; tests for presence of tuberculin
PPRF	paramedian pontine reticular formation
PRPP	phosphoribosyl pyrophosphate
PSA	prostate-specific antigen
PSVT	paroxysmal supraventricular tachycardia
PT	prothrombin time
PTH	parathyroid hormone
PTT	partial thromboplastin time
PTU	propylthiouracil

PUD	peptic ulcer disease
PYR test	L-pyrrolidonyl-beta-naphthylamide test
PZI	protamine zinc insulin
RBC	red blood cell
RDW	red blood cell distribution width index
REM	rapid eye movement
RER	rough endoplasmic reticulum
RES	reticular endothelial system
RLQ	right lower quadrant
RNA	ribonucleic acid
RPF	renal plasma flow
RPGN	rapidly progressive glomerulonephritis
rRNA	ribosomal ribonucleic acid
RSV	respiratory syncytial virus
RV	residual volume
RVH	right ventricular hypertrophy
SA	sinoatrial
SCID	severe combined immunodeficiency disease
SER	smooth endoplasmic reticulum
SES	socioeconomic status
SIADH	syndrome of inappropriate antidiuretic hormone
SIDS	sudden infant death syndrome
SLE	systemic lupus erythematosus
snRNA	small nuclear RNA
SR	sarcoplasmic reticulum
ss	single strand
SSRI	serotonin selective reuptake inhibitor
STD	sexually transmitted disease
SVC	superior vena cava
TAG	triacylglycerol
TAT	thematic apperception test
TB	tuberculosis
TCA	tricarboxylic acid
TCAD	tricyclic antidepressant
TCR	T-cell receptor
TD$_{50}$	median toxic dose
THF	tetrahydrofolate
TIA	transient ischemic attack
TIBC	total iron-binding capacity
TFIID	transcription factor IID
TLC	total lung capacity
Tm	transport maximum
TNF	tumor necrosis factor

TPP	thiamine pyrophosphate
TPR	total peripheral resistance
TRH	thyrotropin-releasing hormone
tRNA	transfer ribonucleic acid
TSH	thyroid-stimulating hormone
TTP	thrombotic thrombocytopenic purpura
TXA$_2$	thromboxane A$_2$
UMN	upper motor neuron
UMP	uridine monophosphate
USMLE	United States Medical Licensing Examination
UTI	urinary tract infection
VC	vital capacity
VIP	vasoactive intestinal peptide
VLDL	very low density lipoprotein
VMA	vanillylmandelic acid
Vmax	maximum velocity
VPL	ventroposterolateral
VPM	ventroposteromedial
V/Q	ventilation-perfusion
VSD	ventricular septal defect
V$_T$	tidal volume
WBC	white blood count

Anatomic Sciences

GROSS ANATOMY

What gland is found in the muscular triangle of the neck?

Thyroid gland

Is an *afferent* or *efferent* pupillary defect described as B/L pupillary constriction when light is shined in the *unaffected* eye and B/L para-doxical dilation when light is shined in the *affected* eye?

Afferent pupillary defect (CN II lesion); in an **efferent** pupillary defect (CN III), B/L **constrict** when light is shined in the unaffected eye and consentual pupil constriction occurs when light is shined in the affected eye.

What is the name of the spinal cord passing within the subarachnoid space and forming the spinal nerves that exit the lumbar and sacral foramina?

Cauda equina

Name the laryngeal muscle described by the following:

Pulls the arytenoids cartilages closer to the thyroid, relaxing the vocal ligaments and thereby decreasing the pitch

Thyroarytenoid muscles

Tenses the vocal ligaments, increasing the distance between the cartilages, thereby increasing the pitch

Cricothyroid muscles

Adducts the vocal ligaments, closes the air passageway during swallowing, and allows phonation	Lateral cricoarytenoid muscles
Only muscle to abduct the vocal cords	Posterior cricoarytenoid muscles
Where does the parotid (Stensen's) duct enter the oral cavity?	Opposite the second upper molar tooth

From what aortic arch are the following structures derived?

Common and internal carotid arteries	Third aortic arch
Degenerates	Fifth
Stapes artery	Second
Maxillary artery	First
Arch of the aorta and right subclavian artery	Fourth
Right and left pulmonary arteries and the ductus arteriosus	Sixth

MS CARD is my mnemonic for the aortic arch derivatives

What abdominal muscle contributes to the anterior layer of the rectus sheath, forms the inguinal ligament, and in men gives rise to the external spermatic fascia of the spermatic cord?	External abdominal oblique

Name the compartment of the lower extremity and the nerve based on its movements.

Adduct the thigh and flex the hip	Medial compartment of the thigh, obturator nerve
Plantar flex the foot, flex the toes, and invert the foot	Posterior compartment of the leg, tibial nerve
Dorsiflex the foot, extend the toes, and invert the foot	Anterior compartment of the leg, deep peroneal nerve
Flex the hip and extend the knee	Anterior compartment of the thigh, femoral nerve
Extend the hip and flex the knee	Posterior compartment of the thigh, tibial nerve
Plantar flex the foot and evert the foot	Lateral compartment of the leg, superficial peroneal nerve

What are the five branches of the posterior cord of the brachial plexus?

STARS
1. Upper **S**ubscapularis
2. **T**horacodorsal
3. **A**xillary
4. **R**adial
5. Lower **S**ubscapularis

Name the correct artery.

The *right* recurrent laryngeal nerve passes around it.	Right brachiocephalic artery
The *left* recurrent laryngeal nerve passes around it.	Arch of the aorta
The inferior mesenteric artery drains into it.	The splenic vein

Are the quadrate and caudate lobes of the liver *functionally* part of the left or right lobe?

Functionally they are part of the **left** lobe of the liver because they receive their blood supply from the left hepatic artery. **Anatomically** they are considered part of the **right** lobe of the liver.

What bones make up the acetabulum?

Pubis, ilium, and ischium

What is the anatomic positioning of the right and left gastric nerve plexus of the esophagus as they pass through the diaphragm?

LARP: Left goes **A**nterior and **R**ight goes **P**osterior (because of the rotation of the gut; remember your embryology!)

What vessel is lacerated in an *epidural* hematoma?

Middle meningeal artery

True or false? Below the arcuate line, all the aponeurotic fibers run anterior to the rectus abdominis.

True

What ocular muscle

Adducts the eyeball and is involved in horizontal conjugate gaze?

Medial rectus (CN III)

Elevates and adducts the eyeball?

Superior rectus (CN III)

Depresses and abducts the eyeball?

Superior **O**blique (CN IV)

Elevates and abducts the eyeball?

Inferior **O**blique (CN III)

***Ab*ducts the eyeball and is involved in horizontal conjugate gaze?**

Lateral **r**ectus (CN VI)

Depresses and adducts the eyeball?

Inferior rectus (CN III)
(LR6 SO4)3

Which muscles of the eye are under parasympathetic control?

Constrictor pupillae and ciliary muscles

Which direction does the uvula deviate in a *left* vagus nerve lesion?

A **left** CN X lesion results in the uvula deviating to the **right**. (Uvula points **away** from the affected side.)

Is a *subdural* hematoma an arterial or venous bleed?

Subdural hematoma is a rupture of the cerebral **veins** where they enter the superior sagittal sinus.

Which CNs are found in the midline of the brainstem?

CN I, II, III, VI, and XII
Add 1 + 1 = 2, 1 + 2 = 3, 1 + 2 + 3 = 6, 1 + 2 + 3 + 6 = 12

What muscles insert in or on the intertubercular groove of the humerus?

"**L**ady between two **M**ajors": latissimus dorsi, pectoralis major, and teres major

What nerve supplies taste sensation to the anterior two-thirds of the tongue?

Chorda tympani of CN VII

What part of the heart forms

The right border?

Right atrium

Left border?

Left ventricle and auricle of left atrium

Apex?

Tip of the left ventricle

Base?

Left atrium and tip of the right atrium

Superior border?

Conus arteriosus of the right ventricle and right and left auricles

Anterior wall?

Right ventricle

Posterior wall?

Left atrium

Diaphragmatic wall?

Left ventricle and tip of right ventricle

What nerves carry the sensory and motor components of the *blink reflex*?

CN **V1** carries the **sensory** and CN **VII** carries the **motor** component of the blink reflex.

What muscle keeps the stapes taut against the oval window?

Stapedius muscle

Name the components of the femoral canal, working laterally to medially.

NAVEL: Femoral **N**erve, **A**rtery, **V**ein, **E**mpty space, and **L**ymphatics/**L**acunar ligament

What muscle is most superior in the orbit?

Levator palpebrae superioris

What portion of the pericardium adheres to the tunica adventitia of the great vessels?

Fibrous pericardium

What two veins form the portal vein?

The superior mesenteric vein and the splenic vein (after it receives the inferior mesenteric vein) join to form the portal vein.

What CNs are responsible for the sensor and motor components of the light reflex?

CN **II** is the **sensory** limb and CN **III** is the **motor** component through parasympathetic stimulation.

Arrange the following layers in the correct sequence through which a needle must pass in a lumbar puncture.

During a lumbar puncture the needle passes through the *interlaminar space* in the midline of *L3–L4*, with the tip of the *iliac crest* in the *flexed* position as the landmark.
Order of puncture:

Skin
Subarachnoid space

1. Skin
2. Superficial fascia

Interspinous ligament
Dura mater
Deep fascia
Epidural space
Superficial fascia
Interlaminar space
Supraspinous ligament
Arachnoid mater

3. Deep fascia
4. Supraspinous ligament
5. Interspinous ligament
6. Interlaminar space
7. Epidural space
8. Dura mater
9. Arachnoid mater
10. Subarachnoid space.

(They ask this in some variation every year, so know it.)

What ocular ganglion is affected if the pupil on the affected side *sluggishly* responds to *light* with *normal accommodation*?

Ciliary ganglion producing a tonic pupil

What is the name for the most prominent spinous process?

Vertebra prominens (C7 in 70% of cases, C6 in 20%, T1 in 10%)

What muscles make up the rotator cuff?

SITS—Subscapularis, **I**nfraspinatus, **T**eres minor, **S**upraspinatus

What is the function of white rami communicantes?

They are preganglionic sympathetic axons. They are white because they are myelinated.

What muscle or muscles are innervated by the following nerves?

    Suprascapular nerve

Supraspinatus and infraspinatus

    Upper subscapularis nerve

Subscapularis

    Thoracodorsal nerve

Latissimus dorsi

    Long thoracic nerve

Serratus anterior

**What nerve is associated
with the following
functions?**

Flex the wrist and digits,
pronate the wrist and
the LOAF (Lumbricales,
Opponens pollicis,
Abductor pollicis
brevis, Flexor pollicis
brevis) muscles of the
hand

Median nerve

Flex the shoulder, flex
the elbow, and supinate
the elbow

Musculocutaneous nerve

Innervation of the flexor
carpi ulnaris, flexor digiti
profundus (pinky and
ring fingers), and the
intrinsic muscles of the
hand

Ulnar nerve

Supinate the wrist,
extend the wrist and
digits, extend the
shoulder and elbow

Radial nerve

**What abdominal muscle
runs horizontally,
contributes to the posterior
rectus sheath, and
contributes to form the
conjoint tendon?**

Transverse abdominis

**Which CNs act as the
sensory and motor
components of the *gag
reflex*?**

The **sensory** limb is via **CN IX,** and the
motor limb is from **CN X**.

Which kidney is lower? Why?

The right kidney is lower in the abdominal cavity because of the amount of space the liver occupies.

What two regions of the vertebral column are considered primary curvatures?

Thoracic and sacral

What vein drains the lower third of the thoracic wall?

Hemiazygous vein

At what point does the axillary artery become the brachial artery?

When it crosses the teres major

What direction would the tongue protrude in a *left* CN XII lesion?

Left CN XII lesion would result in the tongue pointing to the **left** (points **at** the affected side).

At what vertebral level does the common carotid artery bifurcate?

C4 (the upper border of the thyroid cartilage)

True or false? Males are more likely to develop femoral hernias than females.

False. Females are more likely to develop femoral hernias then males (remember **F**emale's **F**emoral).

In what compartment of the thigh is the profundus femoris artery found?

Anterior compartment (it's the blood supply to the posterior compartment)

Where is the cupola of the lung in relation to the subclavian artery and vein?

The cupola of the lung is **posterior** to the subclavian artery and vein. It is the reason one must be cautious when performing subclavian venipuncture.

True or false? The first cervical vertebra has no vertebral body.

True. The odontoid process of C2 acts as the vertebral body of C1 allowing *lateral rotation* of the head.

What is the largest muscle in the body?

Gluteus maximus

At what vertebral levels does the *aortic arch* begin and end?

It both begins and ends at T4 (sternal angle [of Louis]).

What artery travels with the following veins?

   Great cardiac vein

Left anterior descending artery

   Middle cardiac vein

Posterior interventricular artery

   Small cardiac vein

Right coronary artery

The ophthalmic artery is a branch of what vessel?

Internal carotid artery

What structure or structures cross the diaphragm at

   T8 level?

IVC

   T10 level?

Esophagus and esophageal nerve plexus (CN X)

   T12 level?

Aorta, azygos vein, and thoracic duct
Remember: 1 at T8, 2 at T10, and 3 at T12

Is the carotid sinus sensitive to pressure or oxygen?

The carotid sinus is a pressure-sensitive (low) receptor, while the carotid body is an oxygen-sensitive (low) receptor. (Remember "**Sinus Pressure**").

What nerve or nerves supply general sensation and taste to the posterior third of the tongue?

CN XI and X

Which muscle of the eye is under sympathetic control?

Dilator pupillae muscle

True or false? both the left and right lungs have an oblique fissure?

True. on the **right** lung the *oblique fissure* divides the *middle* from the *inferior* lobe and the *horizontal fissure* further divides the *middle* from the *upper* lobe. On the **left** the *oblique* divides the *superior* from the *inferior* lobe.

What are the three branches of the lateral cord of the brachial plexus?

1. Lateral pectoral
2. Lateral head of the median
3. Musculocutaneus

What is the major difference between the veins in the face and the veins in the rest of the body?

There are no valves and no smooth muscle in the walls of the veins in the face.

Name the bony articulations of the following sites. Be specific.

    Shoulder

Clavicle, acromion, and glenoid fossa of the scapula and the humerus

    Elbow

Humerus with ulna (major) and radius (minor)

    Wrist

Radius with scaphoid and lunate and ulna with triquetrum and pisiform (Remember, for major articulations, wrist/radius and humerus/ulna = elbow)

What is the only laryngeal muscle innervated by the external laryngeal nerve?

Cricothyroid muscle; all other laryngeal muscles are innervated by the recurrent laryngeal nerve.

What seven structures are found in more than one mediastinum?

Esophagus, SVC, vagus nerve, azygos vein, thoracic duct, thymus, and phrenic nerve

How many bronchopulmonary

There are **10** bronchopulmonary segments on the **right** and **8** on the **left**.

segments are on the right lung? Left lung?

The duodenal–jejunal flexure is suspended from the posterior abdominal wall by what?

Ligament of Treitz

What is the only tongue muscle innervated by CN X?

Palatoglossus muscle is innervated by **CN X;** all other tongue muscles are innervated by CN XII.

What abdominal muscle runs in a posteroinferior direction, splits to contribute to the rectus sheath, contributes to the formation of the conjoint tendon, and in men gives rise to the middle spermatic fascia and the cremasteric muscle of the spermatic cord?

Internal abdominal oblique

What are the five branches of the superior mesenteric artery?

Inferior pancreaticoduodenal, middle colic, right colic, ileocolic, and 10 to 15 intestinal arteries

What spinal nerves contribute to the pelvic splanchnic (parasympathetic) nerves that innervate the detrusor muscle of the urinary bladder?

S2, S3, S4—keeps the pee-pee off the floor!

What connects the third and the fourth ventricles?

Cerebral aqueduct

What nerve and artery could be affected in a _humeral neck_ fracture?

Axillary nerve and posterior humeral artery

What type of hernia is described as passing through the deep lateral ring of the inguinal canal?

Indirect hernia passes **in** the inguinal canal; a **direct** hernia passes **directly** through Hesselbach's triangle.

What two vessels come together to form the external jugular vein?

1. Posterior auricular vein
2. Posterior division of the retromandibular vein

What is the only vein in the body with a high O_2 content?

The pulmonary vein, which carries oxygenated blood from the lung to the left atrium.

What are the three branches of the celiac trunk?

The left gastric, splenic, and common hepatic arteries

What region of the pharynx does the eustachian tube enter?

Nasopharynx

What is the only muscle of the soft palate that is innervated by CN V3?

The tensor veli palatine is innervated by the mandibular division of the trigeminal nerve; all others are innervated by CN X.

How many pairs of spinal nerves exit from the spinal cord?

31 pairs

What artery turns into the dorsalis pedis when it crosses the extensor retinaculum?

Anterior tibial artery

What is the term for pupils that react *normally* to *accommodation* but have bilateral loss of constriction in response to *light*?

Argyll Robertson pupils

What connects the lateral ventricles to the third ventricle?

Foramen of Monro

What nerve supplies *general* sensation to the anterior two-thirds of the tongue?

Lingual nerve of CN V3

What type of pleura is adherent to the surface of the organ?

Visceral pleura

What artery supplies the left ventricle, left atrium, and interventricular septum?

Left coronary artery

Where are the tonsillar tissues?

Waldeyer's ring

What is the name of the superficial *subcutaneous* fascia of the abdomen containing *fat*?

Camper's fascia; Scarpa's fascia is devoid of fat. (Remember campers are **fat**.)

What are the three anatomic characteristics that differentiate the large bowel from the small bowel and the rectum?

1. Tinea coli
2. Haustra
3. Epiploic appendages

What area of the posterior aspect of the eye has no photoreceptors?

The optic disk is the blind spot.

At the level of rib 6, the internal thoracic artery divides into what two arteries?

Musculophrenic and superior epigastric arteries

What is the name of inflammation of the prepatellar bursa?

Housemaid's knee

What nerve roots constitute the cervical plexus?

C1 through C4

Name the compartment of the mediastinum associated with the following thoracic structures:

Heart and pericardium	Middle
Descending aorta	Posterior
Thymus	Superior and anterior
Phrenic nerve	Superior and middle
Esophagus	Superior and posterior
Trachea	Superior
Ascending aorta	Middle
Thoracic duct	Superior and posterior
Azygos vein	Superior and posterior
SVC	Superior and middle
Splanchnic nerves	Posterior
Aortic arch	Superior
IVC	Middle
Vagus nerve	Posterior
Brachiocephalic vein	Superior
Pulmonary artery and veins	Middle
Left common carotid artery	Superior
Left subclavian artery	Superior

What is the only organ in the body supplied by preganglionic sympathetic fibers?

Adrenal medulla

The *left* subclavian artery is a branch of what artery?

The **left** is a branch of the **aortic arch,** while the **right** is a branch of the **brachiocephalic trunk**.

What are the four muscles of mastication?

1. Masseter
2. Temporalis
3. Medial pterygoid
4. Lateral pterygoid

With what thoracic vertebra or vertebrae does rib 7 articulate?

Rib 7 articulates with T7 and T8. Each rib articulates with the corresponding numerical vertebral body and the vertebral body **below it**.

What are the three branches of the inferior mesenteric artery?

Left colic, superior rectal, and sigmoidal arteries

What is the only valve in the heart with two cusps?

Mitral (bicuspid) valve

What are five clinical signs of portal HTN?

Caput medusa, internal hemorrhoids, esophageal varices, retroperitoneal varices, and splenomegaly

What three muscles constitute the erector spinae?

1. **I**liocostalis
2. **L**ongissimus
3. **S**pinalis
("**I L**ove **S**cience" muscles)

What nerve is compromised in carpal tunnel syndrome?

Median nerve

What vascular injury may result from a supracondylar fracture of the femur?

The popliteal artery, the deepest structure in the popliteal fossa, risks injury in a supracondylar fracture of the femur.

What nerve and artery could be affected in a *midshaft humeral* fracture?

Radial nerve and the profunda brachii artery

Name the 10 retroperitoneal organs.

1. **D**uodenum (all but the first part)
2. Ascending **C**olon
3. **U**reters
4. **P**ancreas
5. **S**upra renal glands (adrenals)
6. **D**escending colon
7. **A**orta
8. **K**idneys
9. **R**ectum
10. **I**VC

D CUPS DAKRI is the mnemonic, everything else is covered with peritoneum

Ventral rami of what cervical nerves constitute the phrenic nerve?

C3, C4, and C5 keep the diaphragm alive!

What is the region of the fallopian tube where fertilization most commonly occurs?

Ampulla

What foramen must be traversed for entry into the lesser peritoneal sac?

Foramen of Winslow

Name the structure that enters or exits the following foramina:

Foramen magnum

CN XI, vertebral arteries

Foramen spinosum

Middle meningeal artery

Foramen rotundum

CN V2

Foramen ovale

CN V3 and the lesser petrosal nerve

Jugular foramen	CN IX, X, and XI; sigmoid sinus
Carotid canal	Internal carotid artery and sympathetic plexus
Stylomastoid foramen	CN VII
Hypoglossal canal	CN XII
Internal auditory meatus	CN VII and VIII
Optic canal	CN II and ophthalmic artery
Cribriform plate	CN I
What vessel can be found atop the scalene anterior?	Subclavian vein
What component of the corneal reflex is lost in a CN VII deficit?	Motor aspect
A motor lesion to the *right* CN V results in deviation of the jaw to which side?	A **right** CN V lesion results in weakened muscles of mastication, and the jaw deviates to the **right.**
What two arteries join to form the superficial and deep palmar arches of the hand?	Ulnar and radial arteries (ulnar is the main supplier)
What two ligaments of the uterus are remnants of the gubernaculum?	Round and ovarian ligaments

What segments of the lumbosacral plexus form the following nerves?

Tibial nerve	L4 to S3
Common peroneal nerve	L4 to S3
Femoral nerve	L2 to L4

Obturator nerve	L2 to L4 (L2 to L4, thigh; L4 to S3, leg)
What three structures are in contact with the left colic flexure? With the right colic flexure?	**Left:** stomach, spleen, and left kidney; **right:** liver, duodenum, and right kidney
What three muscles constitute the pes anserinus?	1. Sartorius 2. Gracilis 3. Semitendinous
What is the only *pharyngeal* muscle *not* innervated by CN X?	Stylopharyngeus muscle is innervated by CN IX; all other pharyngeal muscles are innervated by CN X.
What vessels carry *deoxygenated* blood into the lungs from the right ventricle?	The right and left pulmonary **arteries,** the only arteries that carry deoxygenated blood
Fracture of the fibular neck, resulting in foot drop, is an injury of what nerve?	Common peroneal nerve
What vein is formed by the union of the right and left brachiocephalic veins?	Superior vena cava
If inserting a needle to perform a pleural tap or insertion of a chest tube, do you use the inferior or the superior border of a rib as your landmark? Why?	The **superior border** of the inferior intercostal rib is your landmark for a pleural tap because *along the inferior border* of each rib is the **neurovascular bundle,** and you would risk injury if you went below the rib.
What muscle laterally rotates the femur to unlock the knee?	Popliteus
What chamber of the eye lies between the iris and the lens?	Posterior chamber

What artery supplies the right atrium, right ventricle, sinoatrial and atrioventricular nodes?	Right coronary artery
What four branches of the brachial plexus arise prior to the first rib?	1. Dorsal scapular 2. Suprascapular 3. Long thoracic 4. Nerve to subclavius
What vertebral level is marked by the xiphoid process?	T9

What lower extremity nerve is described by the following motor loss?

Loss of eversion; inversion, dorsiflexion, and plantarflexion of the foot	Common peroneal nerve
Loss of flexion of the knees and toes, plantarflexion, and weakened inversion	Tibial nerve
Loss of knee extension, weakened hip flexion	Femoral nerve
Loss of abduction of the hip resulting in Trendelenburg gait	Superior gluteal nerve
Loss of flexion of the knee and all function below the knee, weakened extension of the thigh	Sciatic nerve
Loss of adduction of the thigh	Obturator nerve

What nerve lesion presents with ape or simian hand as its sign?

Median nerve lesion

What muscle acts in all ranges of motion of the arm?

Deltoid

What is the first branch of the abdominal artery?

Inferior phrenic artery

What vessel does the *right* gonadal vein drain into?

The **right** gonadal vein drains into the **inferior vena cava** directly, and the **left** gonadal vein drains into the **left renal vein**.

What two muscles do you test to see whether CN XI is intact?

Trapezius and sternocleidomastoid

What two CNs are responsible for the carotid body and sinus reflexes?

CN IX and X

At what vertebral level does the trachea bifurcate?

T4 vertebral level posteriorly and anteriorly at the sternal angle (angle of Louis).

What is the function of the arachnoid granulations?

Resorb CSF into the blood

Damage to what nerve will give you winged scapula?

Long thoracic nerve. To avoid confusing **long** thoracic nerve and **lateral** thoracic artery: *long* has an n for nerve; *lateral* has an a for artery.

What portion of the intervertebral disk is a remnant of the notochord?

Nucleus pulposus

What component of the pelvic diaphragm forms the rectal sling (muscle of continence)?

Puborectalis

What are the five branches of the median cord of the brachial plexus?

Four **M**s and a **U**
1. **M**edian
2. **M**edial antebrachial
3. **M**edial pectoral
4. **M**edial brachial cutaneus
5. **U**lnar

What bone houses the ulnar groove?

Humerus (between the medial epicondyle and the trochlea)

What CN is associated with the sensory innervation of

Nasopharynx?

Maxillary division of CN V and glossopharyngeal nerves

Oropharynx?

Glossopharyngeal nerve

Laryngopharynx?

Vagus nerve

What protective covering adheres to the spinal cord and CNS tissue?

Pia mater

What is the name of the urinary bladder where the ureters enter and the urethra exits?

Urinary trigone

What is the term when the brachial artery is compressed, resulting in *ischemic contracture* of the hand?

Volkmann's contracture

What attaches the cusps of the valves to the papillary muscles in the heart?

Chordae tendineae

What is the lymphatic drainage of the pelvic organs?

Internal iliac nodes

What bursa is inflamed in clergyman's knee?	Infrapatellar bursa
What muscle is the chief flexor of the hip?	Psoas major
What component of the ANS, when stimulated, results in bronchoconstriction?	**Parasympathetic** stimulation, via the vagus nerve, results in **bronchoconstriction,** whereas **sympathetic** stimulation results in **bronchodilation.**
What muscles in the hand *ad*duct the fingers?	The **P**almar interosseus **AD**ducts, whereas the **D**orsal interosseus **AB**ducts (**PAD** and **DAB**)
What type of cerebral bleed is due to a rupture of a *berry aneurysm* in the circle of Willis?	Subarachnoid hematoma

What are the five terminal branches of the facial nerve?

1. **T**emporal
2. **Z**ygomatic
3. **B**uccal
4. **M**andibular
5. **C**ervical

(**T**wo **Z**ebras **B**it **M**y **C**lavicle.)

What structure of the knee is described thus?

C-shaped shock absorber; aids in attachment of the tibia to the femur via the medial collateral ligament	Medial meniscus
Prevents posterior displacement and has medial-to-lateral attachment on the tibia	Posterior cruciate ligament
Prevents adduction	Lateral collateral ligament

Prevents anterior displacement and has lateral-to-medial attachment on the tibia	ACL
Prevents abduction	Medial collateral ligament
What branches of CN X are the sensory and motor components of the *cough reflex*? Be specific.	The **sensory** component is through the **superior laryngeal nerve,** and the **motor** limb is via the **recurrent laryngeal nerve**.
What nerves provide sensory innervation *above* the vocal cords? *Below* the vocal cords?	The **internal laryngeal nerve** supplies sensory information from **above** the vocal cords while the **recurrent laryngeal nerve** supplies sensory information **below**.

EMBRYOLOGY

From what pharyngeal groove is the *external auditory meatus* derived?	First pharyngeal groove; all others degenerate.
What embryonic structure forms the adult male structure?	
Corpus cavernosus, corpus spongiosum, and glans and body of the penis	Phallus
Scrotum	Labioscrotal swelling
Urinary bladder, urethra, prostate gland, bulbourethral gland	Urogenital sinus
Testes, seminiferous tubules, and rete testes	Gonads
Ventral part of the penis	Urogenital folds

Gubernaculum testes	Gubernaculum
Epididymis, ductus deferens, seminal vesicle, and ejaculatory duct	Mesonephric duct
Which PG is associated with maintaining a PDA?	PGE and intrauterine or neonatal asphyxia maintain *patency* of the ductus arteriosus. Indomethacin, ACh, and catecholamines promote **closure** of the ductus arteriosus.
When does the primitive gut herniate out of the embryo?	6 weeks
When does it go back into the embryo?	10 weeks
What results when the *palatine* prominences fail to fuse with the other side?	Cleft palate
What is the term for a direct connection between the intestine and the external environment through the umbilicus because the vitelline duct persists?	Vitelline fistula
Where do the primordial germ cells arise?	From the wall of the **yolk sac**
What disorder is due to a 5-α-reductase deficiency, resulting in testicular tissue and stunted male external genitalia?	Male pseudo-intersexuality (hermaphrodite); these individuals are 46XY.
Does the zygote divide mitotically or meiotically?	The zygote divides **mitotically;** only germ cells divide meiotically.

During what embryonic week does the intraembryonic coelom form?   Third week

Name the *primary vesicle* the following structures are derived from (proencephalon, mesencephalon, or rhombencephalon.

Cerebral hemispheres	Proencephalon
Midbrain	Mesencephalon
Cerebellum	Rhombencephalon
Medulla	Rhombencephalon
Diencephalon	Proencephalon
Metencephalon	Rhombencephalon
Telencephalon	Proencephalon
Thalamus	Proencephalon
Eye	Proencephalon°
Pons	Rhombencephalon
Myelencephalon	Rhombencephalon
Pineal gland	Proencephalon°
Cerebral aqueduct	Mesencephalon
Neurohypophysis	Proencephalon°
Third ventricle	Proencephalon
Hypothalamus	Proencephalon°
Lateral ventricles	Proencephalon

°diencephalon derivative

What malignant tumor of the trophoblast causes high levels of hCG and may occur after a hydatidiform mole, abortion, or normal pregnancy?

Gestational trophoblastic neoplasia (GTN or choriocarcinoma)

What syndrome is due to a deficiency of *surfactant*?

Respiratory distress syndrome; treatment with **cortisol** and **thyroxine** can increase production of surfactant.

How many oogonia are present at birth?

None; they are not formed until a girl reaches puberty.

What right-to-left shunt occurs when the aorta opens into the right ventricle and the pulmonary trunk opens into the left ventricle?

Transposition of the great vessels arises from a failure of the aorticopulmonary septum to grow in a spiral.

What are the adult remnants of the following structures?

Left umbilical vein

Ligament teres

Foramen ovale

Fossa ovale

Right and left umbilical arteries

Medial umbilical ligaments

Ductus arteriosus

Ligamentum arteriosum

Ductus venosus

Ligamentum venosum

Mandibular hypoplasia, down-slanted palpebral fissures, colobomas, malformed ears, and zygomatic hypoplasia are commonly seen in what pharyngeal arch 1 abnormality?

Treacher Collins syndrome

What is the tetrad of tetralogy of Fallot?

SHIP: Shifting of the aorta, **H**ypertrophy of the right ventricle, **I**nterventricular septal defect, **P**ulmonary stenosis

What is the term for the external urethra opening onto the *ventral* surface of the penis?

Hypospadia

What CN is associated with the

    First pharyngeal arch?

CN V

    Second pharyngeal arch?

CN VII

    Third pharyngeal arch?

CN IX

    Fourth pharyngeal arch?

CN X

    Fifth pharyngeal arch?

None; it degenerates.

    Sixth pharyngeal arch?

CN X

What disease results in a failure of neural crest cells to migrate to the myenteric plexus of the sigmoid colon and rectum?

Hirschsprung's disease (colonic gangliosus)

What immunologic syndrome is due to a pharyngeal pouch 3 and 4 failure?

DiGeorge's syndrome

What embryonic structure, around *day 19*, tells the ectoderm above it to differentiate into *neural tissue*?

The notochord

What is the term for failure of the testes to descend into the scrotum?

Cryptorchidism; normally the testes descend into the scrotum within 3 months of birth.

Is a membranous septal defect more commonly interventricular or interatrial?

Membranous septal defects are **interventricular;** a persistent **patent ovale** results in an **interatrial** septal defect.

What pharyngeal pouch and groove persist when a pharyngeal fistula is formed?

The second pharyngeal pouch and groove

How early can a pregnancy be detected by hCG assays in the blood? In urine?

hCG can be detected in the **blood** by day **8** and in the **urine** by day **10**.

From what pharyngeal pouch is the following structure derived?

    Middle ear

First

    Superior parathyroid gland and ultimobranchial body of the thyroid

Fourth

    Inferior parathyroid gland and thymus

Third

    Palatine tonsil

Second
M PITS for pharyngeal pouch derivatives

What is the term for the external urethra opening onto the *dorsal* surface of the penis?

Epispadia

True or false? In females, meiosis II is incomplete unless fertilization takes place.

True. The elimination of the unfertilized egg is menses.

What adult structures are derived from preotic somites?

Muscles of the internal eye

What disorder is associated with jaundice, white stools, and dark urine due to biliary duct occlusion secondary to incomplete recanalization?

Extrahepatic biliary atresia

What hormone, produced by the *syncytiotrophoblast*, stimulates the production of *progesterone* by the corpus luteum?

hCG

How many mature sperm are produced by one type B spermatogonium?

Four

All primary oocytes in females are formed by what age?

They are all formed by the **fifth month** of fetal life.

From what embryonic structure are the following structures derived?

The ascending aorta and the pulmonary trunk

Truncus arteriosus

The sinus venarum, coronary sinus, and the oblique vein of the left atrium

Sinus venosus

The right and left ventricles

Primitive ventricle

The aortic vestibule and the conus arteriosus

Bulbus cordis

The right and left atria

Primitive atrium

After a longstanding left-to-right shunt *reverses*, causing cyanosis, and becomes a *right-to-left shunt*, what is it termed?

Eisenmenger's syndrome

True or false? The thyroid gland is an embryologic foregut derivative.

True. The thyroid gland, the lungs, and the pharyngeal pouches are foregut derivatives that are not a component of the gastrointestinal system.

What embryonic structure forms the following adult structures?

Collecting ducts, calyces, renal pelvis, and ureter

Mesonephric duct (ureteric bud)

Urinary bladder and urethra

Urogenital sinus

External genitalia

Phallus, urogenital folds, and labioscrotal swellings

Nephrons, kidney

Metanephros

Median umbilical ligament

Urachus

True or false? The epithelial lining of the urinary bladder and the urethra are embryologic hindgut derivatives.

True

Name the four ventral mesentery derivatives.

1. The lesser omentum (consisting of the hepatoduodenal and hepatogastric ligaments)
2. Falciform ligament
3. Coronary ligament of the liver
4. Triangular ligament of the liver

Liver is ventral; all other ligaments are dorsal mesentery derivatives.

Projectile *nonbilious* vomiting and a small knot at the right costal margin (olive sign) are hallmarks of what embryonic disorder?

Hypertrophic pyloric stenosis due to hypertrophy of the muscularis externa, resulting in a narrowed pyloric outlet

The separation of 46 homologous chromosomes *without* splitting of the centromeres occurs during what phase of meiosis?

Meiosis I; disjunction *with* centromere splitting occurs during meiosis II.

Blood and its vessels form during what embryonic week?

Third week; they are derived from the wall of the yolk sac.

What embryonic structure forms the adult female structures?

Glans clitoris, corpus cavernosus, and spongiosum

Phallus

Gartner's duct

Mesonephric duct

Ovary, follicles, rete ovarii

Gonads

Uterine tube, uterus, cervix, and upper third of the vagina

Paramesonephric ducts

Labia majora

Labioscrotal swelling

Labia minora

Urogenital folds

Ovarian and round ligaments

Gubernaculum

Urinary bladder, urethra, greater vestibular glands, vagina

Urogenital sinus

What direction does the primitive gut rotate? What is its axis of rotation?

The gut rotates clockwise around the superior mesenteric artery.

What syndrome occurs when a 46XY fetus develops testes and *female* external genitalia?

Testicular feminization syndrome (Dude looks like a lady!)

Preeclampsia in the first trimester, hCG levels above 100,00 mIU/mL, and an enlarged bleeding uterus are clinical signs of what?

Hydatidiform mole

True or false? The foramen ovale closes just prior to birth.

False. It closes just **after** birth because the change in pulmonary circulation causes increased left atrial pressure.

At ovulation, in what stage of meiosis II is the secondary oocyte arrested?

Metaphase II

What is the name for failed recanalization of the duodenum resulting in polyhydramnios, bile-containing vomitus, and a distended stomach?

Duodenal atresia

What remains patent in a hydrocele of the testis, allowing peritoneal fluid to form into a cyst?

A patent processus vaginalis

True or false? The respiratory system is derived from the ventral wall of the foregut.

True. The laryngotracheal (respiratory) diverticulum is divided from the foregut by the tracheoesophageal septum.

What is the name for failure of the allantois to close, resulting in a urachal fistula or sinus?

Patent urachus

What structure is derived from the prochordal plate?	The mouth
What is the only organ supplied by the foregut artery that is of mesodermal origin?	Spleen
What tumor is derived from primitive streak remnants and often contains bone, hair, or other tissue types?	Sacrococcygeal teratoma
What two pathologic conditions occur when the gut does not return to the embryo?	Omphalocele and gastroschisis
True or false? For implantation to occur the zona pellucida must degenerate.	True. Remember, it degenerates 4 to 5 days post fertilization, and implantation occurs 7 days post fertilization!
What results when the *maxillary* prominence fails to fuse with the medial nasal prominence?	Cleft lip
What is the direction of growth for the primitive streak, caudal to rostral or rostral to caudal?	The primitive streak grows **caudal to rostral.**
During what embryonic week do somites begin to form?	Third week
In men, at what embryonic week do the primordial germ cells migrate to the indifferent gonad?	Week four, and they remain dormant there until puberty.

What embryonic week sees the formation of the notochord and the neural tube?

Third week

What right-to-left shunt occurs when only one vessel receives blood from both the right and left ventricles?

Persistent truncus arteriosus

What three embryonic cell layers form the chorion?

1. Cytotrophoblast
2. Syncytiotrophoblast
3. Extraembryonic mesoderm

NEUROSCIENCE

Where are the *preganglionic* neuron *cell bodies*, the CNS or the PNS?

They are in the grey matter of the CNS.

Which three CNs send sensory information to the *solitary nucleus*?

CN VII, IX, and X; taste and general sensation for the tongue is sent to the solitary nucleus.

What syndrome is associated with the following brainstem lesions?

Vertebral artery or anterior spinal artery occlusion, resulting in *contralateral* corticospinal tract and medial lemniscus tract deficits and an *ipsilateral* CN XII lesion

Medial medullary syndrome

***Contralateral* corticospinal and medial lemniscus tract deficits and an *ipsilateral* medial strabismus secondary to a lesion in CN VI**

Medial pontine syndrome

Slow-growing *acoustic neuroma* producing CN VII deficiencies	Pontocerebellar angle syndrome
Occlusion of the PICA, resulting in *ipsilateral* limb ataxia, *ipsilateral* facial pain and temperature loss, *contralateral* pain and body temperature loss, *ipsilateral* Horner's syndrome, and *ipsilateral* paralysis of the vocal cords, palate droop, dysphagia, nystagmus, vomiting, and vertigo	Lateral medullary (Wallenberg's) syndrome
AICA or superior cerebellar artery occlusion, resulting in *ipsilateral* limb ataxia, *ipsilateral* facial pain and temperature loss, *contralateral* loss of pain and temperature to the body, *ipsilateral* Horner's syndrome, *ipsilateral* facial paralysis, and hearing loss	Lateral pontine syndrome
Posterior cerebral artery occlusion resulting in a *contralateral* corticospinal tract signs, *contralateral* corticobulbar signs to the lower face, and *ipsilateral* CN III palsy	Medial midbrain (Weber's) syndrome

What CNs are affected if there is a lesion in

The midbrain?	CN III and IV
The upper medulla?	CN IX, X, and XII

Pontomedullary junction?	CN VI, VII, and VIII
The upper pons?	CN V
What is the only CN nucleus found in the cervical spinal cord?	Accessory nucleus

What component of the trigeminal nuclei

Supplies the muscles of mastication?	Motor nucleus of CN V
Receives sensory input (all but pain and temperature) from the face, scalp, dura, and the oral and nasal cavities?	Spinal trigeminal nucleus
Forms the sensory component of the jaw jerk reflex?	Mesencephalic nucleus

What deep cerebellar nuclei receive Purkinje cell projections in

The flocculonodular lobe?	The lateral vestibular nucleus
The vermis?	The fastigial nucleus
The lateral cerebellar hemispheres?	The interposed nucleus
The intermediate hemispheres?	The dentate nucleus

What is the only *excitatory* neuron in the cerebellar cortex, and what is its neurotransmitter?	The granule cell is the only **excitatory** neuron in the cerebellar cortex, and it uses **glutamate** as its neurotransmitter. All the other cells in the cerebellum are **inhibitory** neurons, and they use **GABA** as their neurotransmitter.

What three CNs are associated with conjugate eye movements?

CN III, IV, and VI

What is the term to describe the soft, flabby feel and diminished reflexes seen in patients with acute cerebellar injury to the deep cerebellar nuclei?

Hypotonia (rag doll appearance)

What bedside test is used to differentiate a dorsal column lesion from a lesion in the vermis of the cerebral cortex?

The Romberg sign is present if the patient **sways or loses balance** when standing with **eyes open**. In a **dorsal column lesion,** patients **sway** with **eyes closed**. (Don't forget this one.)

Which one of the cerebellar peduncles is mainly responsible for *outgoing* (*efferent*) information?

Superior cerebellar peduncle; the **inferior** and the **middle** consist mainly of **incoming** (afferent) tracts and fibers.

What tract carries *unconscious proprioceptive* information from the Golgi tendon organs and muscle spindles to the *cerebellum*, helping monitor and modulate muscle movements?

Lower extremity and lower trunk information travels in the dorsal spinocerebellar tract. The **upper** trunk and extremity information travels in the cuneocerebellar tract. (**Cuneocerebellar** and fasciculus **cuneatus** both apply to **upper** extremities.)

What reflex, seen in lesions of the corticospinal tract, is an *extension* of the great toe with *fanning* the of remaining toes?

The Babinski reflex is present in **UMN lesions**. Muscle **atrophy** due to disuse, **hyperreflexia, spastic paralysis, increased** muscle tone, and **weakness** are commonly seen in UMN lesions.

What is the triad of Horner's syndrome?

Ptosis (eyelid drooping), **miosis** (pupillary constriction), and **anhydrosis** (lack of sweating) occur when the preganglionic sympathetic fibers from T1- to T4 are obstructed.

What component of the inner ear

    Contains *perilymph* and responds to angular acceleration and deceleration of the head?

Semicircular canal

    Contains *endolymph* and responds to head turning and movement?

Semicircular duct

    Contains *endolymph* and gravity receptors monitoring *linear* acceleration and deceleration of the head, noting changes in head position?

Utricle and saccule

What is the name of demyelination of the corticospinal tract and the dorsal column in the spinal cord due most commonly to a vitamin B$_{12}$ deficiency?

Subacute combined degeneration, which is **bilateral below the level of the lesion.**

What encephalopathy causes ocular palsies, confusion, and gait abnormalities related to a lesion in the *mammillary bodies* and/or the *dorsomedial nuclei* of the thalamus?

Wernicke's encephalopathy

Which thalamic nucleus receives auditory input from the inferior colliculus?

MGB

Where are the *postganglionic* neuron cell bodies, the CNS or the PNS?

They are in **ganglia** in the PNS.

What disease is a cavitation of the spinal cord causing bilateral loss of pain and temperature at the level of the lesion?

Syringomyelia

What nucleus of the hypothalamus receives visual input from the retina and helps set the circadian rhythm?

Suprachiasmatic nucleus

Are *white* rami preganglionic or postganglionic fibers?

White rami are **preganglionic** fibers, whereas **grey** rami are **postganglionic** fibers.

What area of the hypothalamus is responsible for recognizing a *decrease* in body temperature and mediates the response to conserve heat?

Posterior hypothalamic zones; lesions here result in poikilothermy (environmental control of one's body temperature).

What CN transmits sensory information from the *cornea*?

CN V1, the **occulomotor** division of the **trigeminal** nerve, is the sensory component of the corneal reflex.

What *preganglionic sympathetic* fibers are responsible for innervating the smooth muscle and glands of the pelvis and the hindgut?

Lumbar splanchnics

Where are the cell bodies for the *DCML* and *spinothalamic* sensory systems?

The **first** sensory neuron is in the **dorsal root ganglia**. It carries **ascending sensory** information in the dorsal root of a spinal nerve, eventually synapsing with **second** sensory neuron. In the **brainstem** (DCML) and the **spinal cord** (spinothalamic) the second neuron cell body sends its axons to synapse in the **thalamus**. The **third** sensory neuron cell body is a thalamic nuclei that sends its fibers to the **primary somatosensory cortex.**

What term describes the reflex that increases the curvature of the lens, allowing *near vision*?

Accommodation

What CN carries *preganglionic parasympathetic* fibers that innervate the viscera of the neck, thorax, foregut, and midgut?

CN X (Remember, the vagus nerve supplies the parasympathetic information from the tip of the pharynx to the end of the midgut and all between.)

What area of the hypothalamus is responsible for recognizing an *increase* in body temperature and mediates the response to dissipate heat?

Anterior hypothalamic zone; lesions here result in *hyperthermia*.

What *excitatory* fibers arise from the *inferior olivary nuclei* on the *contralateral* side of the body?

Climbing fibers;, they are monosynaptic input on **Purkinje cells**. Mossy fibers, also **excitatory,** are axons of all other sources and synapse on **granule cells.**

What four CN carry *preganglionic parasympathetic* fibers?

CN III, VII, IX, and X

Name the form of spina bifida.

Meninges and spinal cord project through a vertebral defect

Meningomyelocele

Meninges project through a vertebral defect

Meningocele

An open neural tube lying on the surface of the back

Myeloschisis

Defect in the vertebral arch	Occulta
	All except occulta cause elevated -α-fetoprotein levels.

Name the thalamic nucleus based on its input and output.

Input from the optic tract; output projects to the primary visual cortex of the occipital lobe	LGB (think EYES)
Input from the trigeminal pathways; output to primary somatosensory cortex of the parietal lobe	Ventral posteromedial nucleus
Input from globus pallidus and the cerebellum; output to the primary motor cortex	Ventral lateral nucleus
Input from medial lemniscus and the spinocerebellar tracts; output to the primary somatosensory cortex	Ventral posterolateral nucleus
Input from globus pallidus and substantia nigra; output to primary motor cortex	Ventral anterior nucleus
Input from the amygdala, prefrontal cortex, and temporal lobe; output to the prefrontal lobe and the cingulated gyrus	Medial nuclear group (limbic system)
Input from inferior colliculus; output to primary auditory cortex	MGB (think EARS)

Input from the mammillary bodies via the mammillothalamic tract and the cingulated gyrus; output to the cingulated gyrus via the anterior limb of the internal capsule	Anterior nuclear group (Papez circuit of the limbic system)
What is the name of a thin brown ring around the outer edge of the cornea, seen in Wilson's disease?	Kayser-Fleischer ring
What do UMNs innervate?	They innervate LMNs.
What area of the brain serves as the major *sensory relay center* for *visual, auditory, gustatory,* and *tactile* information destined for the cerebral cortex, cerebellum, or basal ganglia?	The thalamus (I like to think of the thalamus as the executive secretary for the cerebral cortex. All information destined for the cortex has to go through the thalamus.)
Which of the colliculi help direct the movement of both eyes in a gaze?	Superior colliculus (Remember **S** for **S**uperior and **S**ight). The inferior colliculus processes auditory information from both ears.
How do the corticobulbar fibers of CN VII differ from the rest of the CNs?	Normally corticobulbar fiber innervation of the CNs is bilateral (the LMN receives information from both the left and right cerebral cortex), but with CN VII the LMN of the **upper face** receives **bilateral** input but the **lower facial** LMNs receive only **contralateral** input.
What syndrome is described by a lesion in the angular gyrus (area 39) resulting in alexia, agraphia, acalculia, finger agnosia, and right-left disorientation?	Gerstmann's syndrome; spoken language is usually understood.

How many pairs of spinal nerves are associated with

Cervical vertebrae?

Eight pairs through seven cervical vertebrae.

Thoracic vertebrae?

Twelve pairs through twelve thoracic vertebrae.

Lumbar vertebrae?

Five pairs through five lumbar vertebrae.

Sacral vertebrae?

Five pairs through five sacral vertebrae.

Coccygeal vertebrae?

One pair with three to five coccygeal vertebrae.
Totaling 31 pairs of spinal nerves.

What are the three sites where CSF can leave the ventricles and enter the subarachnoid space? (Name the lateral and the medial foramina.)

Two **L**ateral foramina of **L**uschka and 1 **M**edial foramen of **M**onroe (**L** for **L**ateral and **M** for **M**edial)

What CNs arise from

The midbrain?

CN III and IV

The pons?

CN V, VI, VII, and VIII

The medulla?

CN IX, X, and XII
CN XI arises from the cervical spinal cord.

What disconnect syndrome results from a lesion in the corpus callosum secondary to an infarct in the anterior cerebral artery, so that the person can comprehend the command but not execute it?

Transcortical apraxia; Wernicke's area of the left hemisphere cannot communicate with the right primary motor cortex because of the lesion in the corpus callosum.

True or false? Glucose readily diffuses across the blood-brain barrier.

False. Water readily diffuses across the blood-brain barrier, but glucose requires carrier-mediated transport.

What encapsulated group of nerve endings seen at the muscle-tendon junction *responds to an increase in tension* generated in that muscle? (This is dropping a box that is too heavy to carry.)

Golgi tendon organs are stimulated by **Ib afferent neurons** in response to an **increase** in **force or tension**. The inverse muscle reflex **protects** muscle from being torn; it limits the tension on the muscle.

What chromosome 4, AD disorder is a degeneration of GABA neurons in the striatum of the indirect pathway of the basal ganglia?

Huntington's chorea; patients have chorea, athetoid movements, progressive dementia, and behavioral problems.

What syndrome is described as bilateral lesions of the amygdala and the hippocampus resulting in *placidity, anterograde amnesia, oral exploratory behavior, hypersexuality,* and *psychic blindness*?

Klüver-Bucy syndrome

By asking a patient to close the eyes while standing with feet together, what two pathways are you eliminating from proprioception?

When a patient closes the eyes while standing with feet together, the **visual** and **cerebellar components** of proprioception are removed, so you are **testing the dorsal columns. Swaying with eyes closed** is a **positive** Romberg's sign indicating a lesion in the dorsal columns.

The **cold** water caloric test mimics a brainstem lesion by inhibiting the normal reflex response.

(**COWS: C**old **O**pposite **W**arm **S**ame)

What is the name of *bilateral flaccid paralysis*, *hyporeflexia*, and *hypotonia* due to a *viral* infection of the ventral horn of the spinal cord?

Poliomyelitis; it is a bilateral LMN lesion.

What branch off the vertebral artery supplies

The ventrolateral two-thirds of the cervical spinal cord and the ventrolateral part of the medulla?

Anterior spinal artery

The cerebellum and the dorsolateral part of the medulla?

PICA

What syndrome causes inability to concentrate, easy distractibility, apathy, and regression to an infantile suckling or grasping reflex?

Frontal lobe syndrome (lesion in the prefrontal cortex)

True or false? The presence of PMNs in the CSF is *always* abnormal.

True. Although the CSF normally contains 0 to 4 lymphocytes or monocytes, the presence of PMNs is **always** considered abnormal.

What cells lining the ventricles have cilia on their luminal surface to move CSF?

Ependymal cells

What is the most common site for an aneurysm in cerebral circulation?

The junction where the anterior communicating and anterior cerebral arteries join. As the aneurysm expands, it compresses the fibers from the **upper temporal fields** of the optic chiasm, producing **bitemporal inferior quadrantanopia**.

What fissure of the cerebral cortex runs perpendicular to the lateral fissure and separates the frontal and the parietal lobes?

Central sulcus (sulcus of Rolando)

What is the name of violent projectile movements of a limb resulting from a lesion in the subthalamic nuclei of the basal ganglia?

Hemiballismus

What is the term for the type of pupil seen in *neurosyphilis*, and what ocular reflexes are *lost*?

Argyll Robertson pupils accompany a **loss** of both **direct and consensual light reflexes,** but the **accommodation-convergence reaction** remains **intact.** It can also be seen in patients with pineal tumors or multiple sclerosis.

True or false? *Intrafusal* fibers form muscle spindles.

True. **Muscle spindles** are modified skeletal muscle fibers. They are the **sensory component** of the stretch reflexes.

What Brodmann area is associated with

    Broca's area?

Areas 44 and 45

    Primary auditory cortex?

Areas 41 and 42

    Primary somatosensory cortex?

Areas 1, 2, and 3

    Somatosensory association cortex?

Areas 5 and 7

    Primary motor cortex?

Area 4

    Premotor cortex?

Area 6

    Visual association cortex?

Areas 18 and 19

    Frontal eye fields?

Area 8

Primary visual cortex?	Area 17
Wernicke's area?	Area 22 and occasionally 39 and 40
What is the fluid of the posterior compartment of the eye?	Vitreous humor
What aphasia produces a *nonfluent* pattern of speech with the *ability to understand* written and spoken language seen in lesions in the dominant hemisphere?	Expressive aphasia

In a topographical arrangement of the cerebellar homunculus map, what area or lobe

Controls the axial and proximal musculature of the limbs?	The vermis
Is involved in motor planning?	Lateral part of the hemispheres
Controls balance and eye movements?	Flocculonodular lobe (one of my favorite words in all of medicine!)
Controls distal musculature?	Intermediate part of the hemispheres
What glial cell is derived from mesoderm and acts as a scavenger, cleaning up cellular debris after injury?	**M**icroglia (Microglia and mesoderm both begin with **M**)
What direct-pathway basal ganglia disease is described by masklike facies, stooped posture,	Parkinson's disease (I can't underestimate all of the buzzwords in this question. Remember it.)

**cogwheel rigidity,
pill-rolling tremor at rest,
and a gait characterized by
shuffling and chasing the
center of gravity?**

**What artery supplies most
of the lateral surfaces of the
cerebral hemispheres?**

Middle cerebral artery

**What hypothalamic nucleus
is responsible for the
production of *ADH*?**

Supraoptic nuclei; lesions here result in
diabetes insipidus.

**True or false? High-
frequency sound waves
stimulate hair cells at the
base of the cochlea.**

True. *High-frequency* sound waves
stimulate the hair cells at the **base** of the
cochlea, whereas *low-frequency* sound
waves stimulate hair cells at the **apex** of
the cochlea.

**What nucleus of the
hypothalamus is the *satiety
center*, regulating food
intake?**

Ventromedial nucleus; lesions here result
in **obesity.**

**What cells of the retina sees
in *color* and needs bright
light to be activated?**

Cones (**C** for **c**olor and **c**ones)

**What cell's axons are the
only ones that *leave* the
cerebellar cortex?**

The Purkinje cell

**What splanchnic carries
*preganglionic
parasympathetic* fibers that
innervate the hindgut and
the pelvic viscera?**

Pelvic splanchnics (They all begin with
P.)

**Is nystagmus defined by the
fast or slow component?**

Nystagmus is named by the **fast**
component, which is the **corrective**
attempt made by the cerebral cortex in
response to the **initial slow** phase.

Name the ocular lesion; be specific.

Left optic nerve lesion

Left eye anopsia (left nasal and temporal hemianopsia)

Right calcarine cortex lesion

Left homonymous hemianopsia

A right LGB lesion (in the thalamus)

Left homonymous hemianopsia

Optic chiasm lesion

Bitemporal heteronymous hemianopsia

A right lateral compression of the optic chiasm (as in aneurysms in the internal carotid artery)

Right nasal hemianopsia

Left Meyer's loop lesion of the optic radiations.

Left homonymous hemianopsia
Figure 1–1 shows visual field pathways and defects.

What is the function of the cerebellum?

Planning and **fine-tuning** of voluntary skeletal muscle contractions. (Think coordination.) Remember, the function of the **basal ganglia** is to **initiate gross** voluntary skeletal muscle control.

What is the name for inability to stop a movement at the intended target?

Dysmetria; this is seen in a finger-to-nose test.

If a lesion occurs *before* the onset of puberty and arrests sexual development, what area of the hypothalamus is affected?

Preoptic area of the hypothalamus; if the lesion occurs **after** puberty, amenorrhea or impotence will be seen.

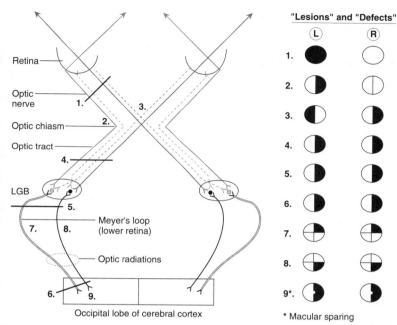

"Lesions" and "Defects"

Figure 1–1.

Lower tract looks to upper quadrant
Upper retina looks to lower quadrant
LGB, lateral geniculate body.

* Macular sparing

Lesion is described by the
Visual Field that is lost.

What sulcus divides the occipital lobe horizontally into a superior cuneus and inferior lingual gyrus?

Calcarine sulcus

Do α- or γ-motor neurons innervate *extrafusal* muscle fibers?

α-Motor neurons innervate **extrafusal** muscle fibers (a motor unit), whereas γ-motor neurons innervate **intrafusal** muscle fibers.

Contracting both medial rectus muscles simultaneously makes the images of near objects remain on the same part of the retina. What term describes this process?

Convergence

Will a *unilateral* lesion in the *spinothalamic tract* result in a contralateral or ipsilateral loss of pain and temperature?

Contralateral. The spinothalamic tract enters the spinal cord and immediately synapses in the dorsal horn, crosses over, and ascends **contralateral** in the spinal cord, brainstem, thalamus, and postcentral gyrus.

What ganglion supplies the *postganglionic parasympathetic* fibers to the *ciliary* muscles of the eye?

Ciliary ganglion

In what tract does *pain, temperature,* and *crude* touch sensory information *ascend* to the *postcentral gyrus* of the parietal lobe?

Spinothalamic tract (anterolateral system)

What CN nucleus receives auditory information from both ears via the cochlear nuclei?

Superior olivary nucleus

What *parasympathetic* nucleus is found on the floor of the fourth ventricle and supplies *preganglionic fibers* innervating the terminal ganglias of the thorax, foregut, and midgut?

Dorsal motor nucleus of CN X

What sensory system is affected in the late spinal cord manifestation of syphilis?

Bilateral degeneration of the **dorsal columns** in the spinal cord secondary to syphilis is known as tabes dorsalis. A high-step gait is seen in patients with tabes dorsalis because of the inability to feel the ground beneath their feet.

What do LMNs innervate?

They innervate skeletal muscle.

What tract carries the *ipsilateral* dorsal column fibers from the *lower limbs* in the spinal cord?

The fasciculus **g**racilis (**G**raceful), which lies **closest** to the midline of the spinal cord.

True or false? CSF is a clear, hypertonic solution with higher concentrations of K$^+$ and HCO$_3^-$, than the serum.

False. CSF is a clear **isotonic** solution with **lower** concentrations of K$^+$ and HCO$_3^-$. It does have higher concentrations of Cl$^-$ and Mg^{2+}.

What type of fiber or fibers are carried in (answer motor, sensory, or both)

Dorsal root?

Sensory

Dorsal rami?

Both

Ventral rami?

Both

Ventral root?

Motor

Dorsal root ganglion?

Sensory

Spinal nerve?

Both

Describe the loss for each of the following in a hemisection of the spinal cord. (Brown–Sáequard syndrome)

Dorsal column tract?

Ipsilateral loss **at and below** the level of the lesion

Corticospinal tract?

Ipsilateral loss **below** the level of the lesion

LMN?

Ipsilateral flaccid paralysis

Spinothalamic tract?

Contralateral loss **below** and **bilateral** loss **at** the level of the lesion

What area of the brain acts as the center for *ipsilateral* horizontal gaze?

PPRF

What aphasia is seen as an inability to comprehend spoken language and speaking in a *word salad*?

Receptive aphasia is due to a lesion in Brodmann areas 22, 39, and 40; generally the patient is **unaware** of the deficit.

What is the function of the basal ganglia?

Initiate and manage **gross** skeletal muscle movement control

What artery is formed by the union of the two vertebral arteries?

The basilar artery is formed at the pontomedullary junction.

What disease is described by bilateral flaccid weakness of the upper limbs (LMN) and bilateral spastic weakness of the lower limbs (UMN) beginning at the *cervical* level of the spinal cord and progressing up or down the cord?

Amyotrophic lateral sclerosis (Lou Gehrig's disease) is a **LMN** lesion **at the level of the lesion** and **UMN** lesion **below the level of the lesion.**

Which dopamine receptor *excites* the direct pathway of the basal ganglia?

D1 receptor; **inhibition** of the direct pathway occurs through the **D2** receptors.

Does the *direct* or *indirect* basal ganglia pathway result in a *decreased* level of cortical excitation?

Although both pathways are associated with disinhibition, the **indirect** basal ganglia pathway is associated with a **decreased** level of cortical excitation.

What fissure of the cerebral cortex separates the frontal and temporal lobes rostrally and partially separates the parietal and temporal lobes?

Lateral fissure (fissure of Sylvius)

What area of the brain acts as the center for *contralateral* horizontal gaze?

Frontal eye field (Brodmann area 8)

In an adult, where does the spinal cord terminate and what is it called?

The conus medullaris terminates at the level of the second lumbar vertebra.

If a patient with a cerebellar lesion has nystagmus, which way is the fast component directed, toward or away from the lesion?

The fast component is directed toward the affected side of a cerebellar lesion.

What area of the limbic system is responsible for attaching *emotional significance to a stimulus*?

Amygdala; it helps imprint an emotional response in memory.

What is the name of the tremor that occurs during movements and is *absent* while the person is *at rest*?

Intention tremor; it is a sign of cerebellar lesions. A tremor at rest (i.e., pill rolling) is seen in basal ganglia lesions.

What is the term for making up stories regarding past experiences because of an inability to retrieve them?

Confabulation; it is commonly seen in Korsakoff's syndrome.

What frontal lobe cortex is associated with organizing and planning the intellectual and emotional aspect of behavior?

Prefrontal cortex; it is in front of the premotor area.

What is the largest nucleus in the midbrain?

The substantia nigra is the largest nucleus in the midbrain. It contains melanin and uses GABA and dopamine as its neurotransmitters.

Where is the lesion that produces these symptoms when a patient is asked to look to the *left*?

***Left* eye can't look to the left**

Left abducens *nerve*

Right eye can't look *left*, *left* eye *nystagmus*, and convergence is intact	**Right** medial longitudinal fasciculus
Neither eye can look *left* with a *slow* drift to the *right*	**Left** abducens *nucleus* or **right** cerebral cortex
What area of the hypothalamus is the *feeding center*?	Lateral hypothalamic zone; lesions here result in *aphagia*. (Notice the difference between the feeding center and the satiety center; they are in different zones.)
In what pathway of the basal ganglia do lesions result in *hyperactive* cortex with *hyperkinetic*, *chorea*, *athetosis*, *tics*, and *dystonia*?	Indirect pathway (Tourette syndrome for example)
What happens to muscle tone and stretch reflexes when there is a LMN lesion?	The **hallmarks** of LMN lesion injury are **absent** or decreased reflexes, muscle **fasciculations, decreased** muscle tone, and muscle **atrophy** (**flaccid paralysis**). Don't forget, LMN lesions are **ipsilateral at the level** of the lesion!
In what pathway of the basal ganglia do lesions result in an *underactive* cortex with *hypokinetic*, *slow*, or absent *spontaneous* movement?	Direct pathway; a good example is Parkinson's disease.
What sided muscle weakness is seen in an UMN corticospinal tract injury *above* the pyramidal decussation?	**Contralateral** muscle weakness when *above* the decussation, whereas an UMN injury *below* the pyramidal decussation results in **ipsilateral** muscle weakness.
What area of the retina consists of only cones and has the greatest visual acuity?	Fovea

What tract carries the *ipsilateral* dorsal column fibers from the *upper limbs* in the spinal cord?

The fasciculus cuneatus

What CNS demyelinating disease is characterized by *diplopia, ataxia, paresthesias, monocular blindness and weakness*, or spastic paresis?

Multiple sclerosis

What part of the ANS (i.e., PNS or CNS) controls the *constriction* of the pupil in response to *light*?

Parasympathetic

With which CN are *preganglionic parasympathetic* axons arising from the *Edinger-Westphal* nucleus associated?

CN III

Ophthalmic artery is a branch of what artery?

Internal carotid artery

What thalamic relay nucleus do the mammillary bodies project to?

The anterior nucleus of the thalamus

What cells contribute to the blood-brain barrier and proliferate in response to CNS injury?

Astrocytes

What causes slow writhing movements (athetosis)?

Hypermyelination of the corpus striatum and the thalamus (seen in cerebral palsy)

What area of the brain is responsible for *emotion, feeding, mating, attention,* and *memory*?

The limbic system

What is the name of the *postganglionic parasympathetic* ganglion that innervates

> **The papillary sphincter and ciliary muscle of the eye?**

Ciliary ganglion. (These fibers are carried in CN III. Remember it like this: -ili- in ciliary ganglion looks like the III of CN III.)

> **The parotid gland?**

The otic ganglion. (These fibers are carried in CN IX. Remember it like this: the -**oti**- is in both **oti**c ganglion and par**oti**d gland.)

> **The submandibular and sublingual glands?**

The submandibular ganglion. (Submandibular ganglion innervates the submandibular gland; easy enough.)

> **The lacrimal gland and oral and nasal mucosa?**

Pterygopalatine ganglion (I remember this as the only ganglion left.)

What neuronal cell bodies are contained in the *intermediate zone of the spinal cord*? (T1–L2)

Preganglionic sympathetic neurons

What limb of the internal capsule is *not* supplied by the middle cerebral artery?

Anterior limb of the internal capsule is supplied by the anterior cerebral artery.

What tract is responsible for *voluntary refined movements of distal extremities*?

Corticospinal tract

Craniopharyngiomas are remnants of what?

Rathke's pouch; they can result in compression of the optic chiasm.

Clarke's nucleus is the second ascending sensory neuron of which spinocerebellar tract?

Dorsal spinocerebellar tract; the **accessory cuneate nucleus** is the second nucleus for the **cuneocerebellar tract**.

Name the *three postganglionic sympathetic ganglia* that receive input from *thoracic splanchnics.*

Celiac, aorticorenal, and superior mesenteric ganglias. (Remember all "Splanchnics" are **S**ympathetic except for the **P**elvic splanchnics, which are **P**reganglionic **P**arasympathetic fibers.)

What is the only CN to arise from the dorsal surface of the midbrain?

CN IV

What basic reflex regulates muscle tone by contracting muscles in *response to stretch* of that muscle?

The myotatic reflex is responsible for the tension present in all **resting muscle.**

Where are the LMN cell bodies of the *corticospinal tract*?

In the ventral horn of the spinal cord. UMN cell bodies are in the precentral gyrus of the frontal lobe.

What nucleus, found in the *intermediate zone of the spinal cord,* sends unconscious proprioception to the cerebellum?

Clarke's nucleus

The vertebral artery is a branch of what artery?

The subclavian artery

What muscle of the middle ear is innervated by the mandibular division of CN V?

Tensor tympani

The fibers of nucleus gracilis and nucleus cuneatus *cross* at the *medullary decussation* and ascend *contralateral* to what thalamic relay nucleus?

VPL nucleus sends its fibers to synapse in the **postcentral gyrus** of the parietal lobe.

What muscle of the middle ear is innervated by CN VII?

The stapedius muscle

What part of the inner ear contains the gravity receptors for changes in the position of the head? — Saccule and utricle

What nucleus supplies the *preganglionic parasympathetic* fibers to the *ciliary* ganglion? — Edinger-Westphal nucleus (via CN III)

What reticular nuclei synthesize serotonin from L-tryptophan and plays a role in mood, aggression, and inducing sleep? — The raphe nuclei

Will a patient with a unilateral lesion in the cerebellum fall toward or away from the affected side? — Patients with unilateral cerebellar lesions fall toward the side of the lesion.

A unilateral lesion in what nucleus will produce ipsilateral paralysis of the *soft palate*? — Nucleus ambiguus, resulting in the uvula deviating *away* from the side of the lesion.

True or false? Neurons in the dorsal horn participate in reflexes. — True. They are the sensory component of a spinal reflex.

What ganglion receives *preganglionic sympathetic* fibers from T1 to L1–2 and innervates smooth muscle, cardiac muscle, glands, head, thoracic viscera, and blood vessels of the body wall and limbs? — Sympathetic chain ganglion

What *preganglionic sympathetic* fibers are — Thoracic splanchnic fibers

responsible for innervating
the foregut and the midgut?

**Does light or darkness
regulate the pineal gland?**

Light regulates the activity of the pineal
gland via the retinal–suprachiasmatic–
pineal pathway.

**Name the three hormones
produced by pinealocytes.**

Melatonin, serotonin, and CCK

**Is the pH of CSF acidotic,
alkalotic, or neutral?**

The pH of CSF is 7.33, acidotic.

**What ascending sensory
system carries joint
position, vibratory and
pressure sensation, and
discriminative touch from
the trunk and limbs?**

The DCML system. (Remember,
everything but pain and temperature.)

**What reflex enables the
eyes to remain focused on
a target while the head is
turning?**

The vestibulo-ocular reflex

**What cells of the retina see
in *black and white* and are
used for night vision?**

Rods

HISTOLOGY

**Name the muscle type
based on these descriptions:**

**_Discontinuous voluntary_
contraction, *multi*nuclear
striated *unbranched*
fibers, actin and myosin
overlapping for banding
pattern, *triadic* T tubules,
troponin and desmin as Z
disc intermediate
filament.**

Skeletal muscles (Fig. 1–2)

Skeletal muscle fiber

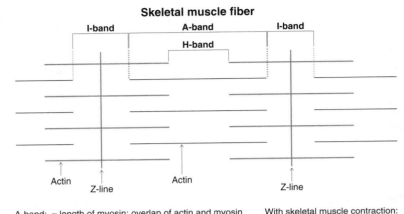

A-band: ≈ length of myosin; overlap of actin and myosin
H-band: Actin to actin ends within a carcomere
I-band: End of myosin to myosin between **2** sarcomeres
Myosin: Thick filament
Actin: Thick filament

With skeletal muscle contraction:
1. H-band and I-bands **shorten**
2. ØΔ in A-band length

Figure I–2.

Continuous involuntary contraction, uninuclear striated branched fibers, actin and myosin overlapping for banding pattern, *dyadic* T tubules, *intercalated discs*, troponin and desmin as a Z disc intermediate filament.	Cardiac muscle
***Involuntary* contraction, uninuclear *nonstriated* fibers, actin and myosin *not forming* banding pattern; *lack* of T tubules, *gap junctions*, and calmodulin.**	Smooth muscle
What segment of the small intestine is associated with *Brunner's glands*?	Duodenum

Who is responsible for passing on mitochondrial DNA genetic disorders?

Mitochondria-linked disorders are always inherited from the **mother**.

What part of a neuron *receives* information?

Dendrites receive information, whereas axons send information.

What type of collagen is associated with the basement membrane?

Type IV collagen

What is the epithelial lining of the *prostatic* portion of the urethra?

Transitional epithelium. The distal portion of the **penile** urethra is composed of *stratified* epithelium.

What cell of the nephron is responsible for *renin* production and secretion?

Juxtaglomerular (JG) cell

What cell surface modification of ependymal cells and respiratory epithelium has a 9 + 2 microtubular configuration and movement as its function?

Cilia

True or false? The following are functions of hepatocytes: protein production, bile secretion, detoxification, conjugation, and lipid storage.

True. (They are quite a busy bunch of cells!)

What substance found in eosinophils is toxic to parasitic worms?

Major basic protein

After fertilization, what cells of the corpus luteum

Secrete progesterone?

Granulose cells secrete progesterone. After fertilization the granulose cells form from follicular cells.

Secrete estrogen?

Theca cells secrete estrogen. After fertilization the theca cells form from the theca interna.

What is the largest organ in the body?

Integument (skin and its derivatives)

On what layer of the epidermis does *all* mitosis occur?

Malpighian layer (made up of the stratum basale and stratum spinosum)

What ribosomal subunit binds first to the mRNA strand?

The small subunit (40S) binds first.

What is the T-cell area of the spleen?

PALS

What element is needed for the proper alignment of tropocollagen molecules?

Copper (Cu^+)

What type of cell surface projection lies on the lateral surface of cells closest to the apex and acts to seal off the outside environment from the rest of the body?

Zonula occludens (tight junctions)

What organelle is responsible for ribosomal RNA synthesis?

Nucleolus. Ribosomal assembly also takes place in the nucleolus.

What sweat gland type is associated with odor production and hair follicles and is found in the axilla?

APocrin**E** glands (**APES** is my memory aid) **A**xilla, **A**reola, and **A**nus all begin with **A. APES** are hairy (associated with hair follicles). They smell (odor production), and if confronted by an **APE,** your **A**drenergic nervous system would be firing (innervation).

What papillae send their senses via chorda tympani of CN VII?

Fungiform papillae

True or false? The portal tract of the liver lobule is the first area to be oxygenated in the liver.

True. (Remember, blood flows from the portal tracts to the central vein, so it is the first area to receive blood and therefore oxygen.)

Match the chromosome and haploid number with the stage of sperm development, spermatid, spermatocyte (primary or secondary), spermatogonia (type A or B):

46/2n (divide meiotically)	Spermatogonia (type A)
46/4n	Primary spermatocyte
23/1n	Spermatid
46/2n (divide mitotically)	Spermatogonia (type B)
23/2n	Secondary spermatocyte

What are the four functions of SER?

Steroid synthesis, drug detoxification, triglyceride resynthesis, and Ca^{2+} handling

Which immunoglobulin is secreted by the plasma cells in the gastrointestinal tract?

IgA

What area of the lymph node is considered the thymic-dependent area?

The inner cortex (paracortex) contains the T cells, so it is considered the thymic-dependent area.

What type of chromatin is transcriptionally *inactive*?

Heterochromatin, the light stuff in the nucleus on an electron microscope image.

Both submandibular and sublingual glands are innervated by CN VII (facial) and produce mucous and serous secretions. Which one mainly produces serous secretions?

Submandibular gland produces mainly **serous** and the *sublingual gland* produces mainly **mucous** secretions.

What is the only neuroglial cell of mesodermal origin?

Microglia. All others are neuroectodermal derivatives.

Where is tropocollagen aggregated to form a collagen fibril?

Outside the cell

What are the four posttranslational modifications done by the Golgi apparatus?

1. Phosphorylation of mannose (lysosomes only)
2. Removal of mannose residues
3. Formation of glycosylate proteins
4. Phosphorylation of sulfate amino acids

What is the epithelial cell lining the nasopharynx?

Stratified squamous nonkeratinized epithelium, which has cilia that beat *toward* the oropharynx.

What are the three epidermal derivatives?

1. Nails
2. Hair
3. Sweat glands (both apocrine and sebaceous)

What are the long microvilli in the inner ear and male reproductive tract called?

Stereocilia

True or false? The central vein of the liver lobule is the first area affected during hypoxia.

True. Blood flows *from* the portal tracts (distal) *to* the central vein (proximal), so it is the first area affected during hypoxia.

What cell of the male reproductive system *produces* testosterone?

Leydig cells produce testosterone. **L**H stimulates **L**eydig cells. (Both start with **L**.)

Myelin is produced by which cells in the PNS? In the CNS?

In the PNS, myelin is produced by Schwann cells, in the CNS by oligodendrocytes.

What cell type of the epidermis functions as antigen-presenting cells?

Langerhans cells (found in the stratum spinosum)

What cell type is found in the peripheral white pulp of the spleen?

B cells are mainly found in the peripheral white pulp and germinal centers in the spleen.

What area of the female reproductive tract is lined by stratified *squamous* epithelium rich in glycogen?

The vagina

What encapsulated lymphoid organ is characterized by presence of Hassall's corpuscles, and absence of germinal centers and B cells?

Thymus gland. (Thymus gland is essential for T cell maturation.)

What cell transports IgA, is secreted by plasma cells, and is in Peyer's patches to the gastrointestinal lumen?

M-cells

What are the cells of the parathyroid gland that produce PTH?

Chief cells

What skin type on the palms and soles is characterized by the absence of hair follicles and presence of stratum lucidum?

Thick skin

What is the name of hydrophilic pores that allow the direct passage of ions and particles between two adjacent cells?

Gap junctions

What type of lysosome is formed when lysosome fuses with a substrate for breakdown?

Secondary lysosome (think of the primary as **inactive** and secondary as **active**)

What cell membrane structure increases the surface area of a cell and has actin randomly assorted within its structure?

Microvillus

What are the four components of the basement membrane?

1. Laminin
2. Heparan sulfate (heparitin sulfate)
3. Fibronectin
4. Type IV collagen

What organelle synthesizes proteins that are intended to stay *within the cell*?

Free polysomes. *Membrane-associated polysomes* are the site of protein synthesis destined to **leave the cell.**

What cell type of the body or fundus of the stomach secretes *IF*?

Parietal cells (Remember, they secrete HCl, too.)

What cell type of the body or fundus of the stomach secretes pepsinogen?

Chief cells

What hormone, produced by the granulose cell, stimulates the endometrium to enter the *proliferative* phase?

Estrogen; the first 14 days of the female reproductive cycle mark the proliferative phase.

What cells of the nephron function as sodium concentration sensors of the tubular fluid?

Macula densa

What type of chromatin is transcriptionally *active*?

Euchromatin, the dark stuff in the nucleus on an electron microscope image.

What cells of the thyroid gland secrete calcitonin?

Parafollicular C cells

True or false? The nucleus is the site of *transcription*.

True. Transcription (conversion of DNA to RNA), as well as replication, occurs in the nucleus.

How many days *after* the LH surge is ovulation?

One day after the LH surge and 2 days after the estrogen peak.

In what layer of the epidermis is melanin transferred from melanocytes to keratinocytes?

Stratum spinosum

What cells of the epidermis, derived from the neural crest, act as mechanoreceptors?

Merkel cells (Merkel's tactile cells)

What substance do the JG cells of the kidney secrete in response to low blood pressure?

Renin

What is the rule of one-third regarding muscle type of the esophagus?

Upper third skeletal muscle, **middle third** both skeletal and smooth muscle, and **lower third** smooth muscle

What papillae are responsible for sweet taste?

Circumvallate papillae

What area of the lymph node contains germinal centers?

The outer cortex contains most of the germinal centers and therefore also most B cells.

True or false? The gallbladder functions to produce bile.

False. The gallbladder does *not produce* bile, but it **concentrates** bile via active sodium transport; water follows the sodium.

True or false? *Depolarization* of the postsynaptic membrane excites the neuron.

True. **Hyperpolarization** inhibits the postsynaptic membrane.

In the alveoli, what cell type is

for gas exchange?

Type I pneumocytes

responsible for producing surfactant?
Type II pneumocytes

part of the mononuclear phagocytic system?
Alveolar macrophages (dust cells)

Which trophoblast layer of the placenta remains until the end of pregnancy?
Syncytiotrophoblast. (The cytotrophoblast gets incorporated into the syncytiotrophoblast.)

What is the first epidermal layer without organelles and nuclei?
Stratum lucidum

What area of the small intestine is characterized by *Peyer's patches*?
Ileum

What lymphoid organ has the following characteristics: outer and inner cortical areas, encapsulation, germinal centers, and high endothelial venules?
Lymph nodes

What area of the nephron is sensitive to the effects of ADH?
Collecting ducts, which make them readily permeable to water reabsorption.

What is the name of RER in neurons?
Nissl substances; there is a great deal of RER in neuron cell bodies, indicating high protein synthesis.

What hormone causes milk letdown?
Oxytocin

What are the three reasons for the effectiveness of the blood-brain barrier?
1. Tight junctions
2. Capillaries that lack fenestration
3. Very selective pinocytosis by the capillaries

What cell type of the epidermis originates from the neural crest?

Melanocytes

If no fertilization occurs, how many days after ovulation does the corpus luteum begin to degenerate?

12 days after ovulation

What area of the spleen consists of splenic cords of Billroth and phagocytoses RBCs?

Red pulp (Remember, **R**ed pulp and **R**BCs begin with **R**.)

What is the name of the protein coat that surrounds the nuclear envelope?

Vimentin

What papillae are touch receptors on the tongue and send their sensations via CN V3 (mandibular division)?

Filiform papillae

What is the most superficial layer of the epidermis?

Stratum corneum (keratinized)

What syndrome is characterized by dynein arm abnormality resulting in chronic sinusitis, recurrent pulmonary infections, and infertility?

Kartagener's syndrome (also known as immotile cilia syndrome)

What are the functions of the zonula occludens and the zonula adherens?

To provide attachment between contiguous cells and to maintain a semipermeable barrier

What is the name of the SER of striated muscle?

Sarcoplasmic reticulum

Where do sperm go for maturation?

Ductus epididymis, which is lined by pseudostratified epithelium with stereocilia.

When is the first arrested stage of development in the female reproductive cycle?

Prophase of meiosis I (between 12th and 22nd week *in utero*)

What is the longest and most convoluted segment of the nephron?

PCT

What cells of the epidermis carry the pigment melanin?

Keratinocytes, the most numerous cells in the epidermis, *carry* **melanin** and *produce* **keratin.**

What segment of the gastrointestinal tract lacks villi, has crypts, and actively transports sodium out of its lumen?

Large intestine. Water is **passively** removed from the lumen.

What two areas of the skin do *not* contain sebaceous glands?

Palms and soles of the feet. Sebaceous glands are associated with hair follicles, which are lacking on the palms and soles of the feet.

Which of the following is *not* part of the *conducting portion* of the respiratory system: trachea, bronchi, alveoli, or larynx?

Alveoli; they are part of the respiratory portion.

Where are the enzymes for the ETC and oxidative phosphorylation found?

The inner membrane of the mitochondria (cristae)

What lymphoid organ is characterized by germinal centers, plasma cells that secrete IgA, and *no* encapsulation?

Peyer's patch

What generate *anterograde* transport of information in a neuron?

Kinesins. Dynein generates **retrograde** transportation of information.

What is the only glycosaminoglycan (GAG) that binds to the linker portion of the proteoglycan?

Hyaluronic acid (all sulfates bind to the core protein)

What cell in bone is a part of the mononuclear phagocytic system?

Osteoclasts

What three factors do Sertoli cells produce for normal *male* development?

Inhibin, müllerian-inhibiting factor, and androgen binding protein

What epidermal layer's function is to release lipids to act as a sealant?

Stratum granulosum

What does the tunica intima of arteries have that veins do not?

An internal elastic lamina

Do the duct or the acini cells of the pancreas secrete HCO_3^-?

Duct cells secrete **HCO_3^-, electrolytes, and water.** The *acini* secrete the **enzymes** necessary for carbohydrate, nucleic acid, protein cleavage, and emulsification of fats.

What cell of the duodenum contains high concentrations of *lysozymes* and has *phagocytic activity*?

Paneth cells

What maintains the osmotic gradient that is critical to the concentrating ability of the kidney?

The *venae recta* maintain the gradient via countercurrent flow.

Are the JG cells of the nephron a part of the afferent or efferent arteriole?

Afferent arteriole

What cell of the duodenum secretes *CCK*?

Entero**e**ndocrine (EE) cells; they also secrete **secretin.**

What are the proteoglycans of cartilage and bone?

Chondroitin sulfate and keratan sulfate

What is the term for the first 3 to 5 days of the female reproductive cycle?

Menses. (**Ovulation** occurs 14 days **before** the **beginning** of menses.)

What is the second arrested stage of development in the female reproductive cycle?

Metaphase of meiosis II (in the oocyte of the graafian follicle)

What ribosomal subunit sizes do eukaryotic cells have?

60S and 40S. The large subunits (60S) are made in the *nucleolus* and the small subunits (40S) are made in the *nucleus*.

What term describes how an action potential is propagated along an axon?

Saltatory conduction

What phase of the female reproductive cycle is 14 days long?

The *secretory phase* is **progesterone**-dependent and 14 days long, whereas the length of the proliferative phase varies.

A single mRNA strand translated by a ribosome is termed what?

Polysome. Ribosomes read from the 5′ to the 3′ end of the mRNA.

What cell is under control of FSH and testosterone; secretes inhibin, MIF, and androgen-binding protein; and phagocytizes the excess cytoplasm of the spermatid?

Sertoli cell

What histone binds two nucleosomes together?

H1 histones

What is the major inorganic component of bone?

Hydroxyapatite

What cells of the adrenal gland are neural crest derivatives?

Chromaffin cells (adrenal medulla)

Where does β-oxidation of very long chain fatty acids begin?

In the peroxisome until it is 10 carbons long; the rest is completed in the mitochondria.

What organelles make ATP, have their own dsDNA, and can synthesize protein?

Mitochondria

Behavioral Sciences

How do delusions, illusions, and hallucinations differ?

Hallucinations are sensory impressions (without a stimulus); illusions are misperceptions of real stimuli; and delusions are false beliefs that are not shared by the culture.

What syndrome is characterized by sweating, insomnia, nausea, diarrhea, cramps, delirium, and general restlessness secondary to MAOI and SSRI in combination?

Serotonin syndrome. It is also associated with high doses and MAOI and synthetic narcotic combinations (Ecstasy). Treatment consists of decreasing SSRI dosage, removing the causative agent, and giving cyproheptadine.

What is the legal age to be deemed competent to make decisions?

18 years old (except if emancipated)

With what stage of sleep is enuresis associated?

Stage 3 and 4 most commonly. It can occur at any stage in the sleep cycle and is usually associated with a major stressor being introduced into the home.

When more than one explanation can account for the end result, what form of bias occurs?

Confounding bias

Increased levels of what neurotransmitter, in the hippocampus, *decrease* the likelihood of learned helplessness?

Increased GABA levels *decrease* the likelihood of learned helplessness.

How do barbiturates affect sleep?

By causing rebound insomnia and decrease in REM sleep

What type of correlation compares two *ordinal variables*?

Spearman correlation

What syndrome is characterized by bilateral medial temporal lobe lesion, placidity, hyperorality, hypersexuality, hyperreactivity to visual stimuli, and visual agnosia?

Klüver-Bucy syndrome

What is the term for having fantasies or dressing in female clothes for sexual arousal by *heterosexual* men?

Transvestite fetishism

What disorder is described as having

**   *Unconscious* symptoms with *unconscious* motivation?**

Somatoform disorder

**   *Conscious* symptoms with *conscious* motivation?**

Malingering

**   *Conscious* symptoms with *unconscious* motivation?**

Factitious disorder

What is the term for the ability of a test to measure something consistently?

Reliability (think of it as "nice grouping" or "precise")

What cerebral vessel size is affected in patients with vascular dementia?

Small to medium-sized cerebral vessels

What is the name of the program that deals with codependency and enabling behaviors for family members of alcohol abusers?

Al-Anon

What level of mental retardation is characterized by

    Needing a highly structured environment with constant supervision?

Profound (I.Q. range < 20)

    Having the ability to communicate and learn basic habits but training is usually not helpful?

Severe (range 20–34)

    Being self-supportive with minimal guidance and able to be gainfully employed (includes 85% of the mentally retarded)?

Mild (50–70)

    Can work in sheltered workshops and learn simple tasks but need supervision?

Moderate (35–49)

Name these *immature* defense mechanisms:

    Taking others' beliefs, thoughts, and external stimuli and making them part of the self. (Hint: if it's done consciously, it is called imitation.)

Introjection (a sports fan is a good example)

    Returning to an earlier stage of development (e.g., enuresis)

Regression

    Inability to remember a known fact (aware of forgetting)

Blocking. (I call it a brain fart!)

Psychic feelings converted to physical symptoms	Somatization
What is the term for ejaculation before or immediately after vaginal penetration on a regular basis?	Premature ejaculation

At what stage of cognitive development (according to Piaget) do children

See death as irreversible?	Concrete operations (6–12 years)
Have abstract thinking?	Formal operations (>12 years)
Lack law of conservation and be egocentric?	Preoperational (2–6 years)
Is it acceptable to lie, even if it protects a colleague from malpractice?	No, it is never acceptable to lie.
What happens to prevalence as duration increases?	Prevalence increases. (Note: Incidence does not change.)
With what stage of sleep are nightmares associated?	REM sleep. Nightmares are frightening dreams that we recall.
What is the statistical term for the proportion of *truly nondiseased persons* in the screened population who are *identified as nondiseased*?	Specificity (it deals with the healthy)

In the elderly, what happens to total sleep time, percentage of REM sleep, and percentage of NREM sleep?

Total and NREM sleep decrease considerably as we age, but REM sleep remains relatively constant (20%) up to age 80, then begins to decline.

What happens to dopamine levels when we awaken?

Dopamine levels rise with waking; dopamine is associated with wakefulness.

What is the primary risk factor for suicide?

Previous suicide attempt

What is defined as a general *estimate* of the functional capacities of a human?

IQ

What dementia is associated with dilated ventricles with diffuse cortical atrophy, decreased parietal lobe blood flow, and a decrease in *choline acetyl transferase* activity?

These are the gross pathologic changes associated with Alzheimer's disease.

What is the term for a deficiency or absence of sexual fantasies or desires?

Hypoactive sexual desire disorder

What phobia is described as the fear of open spaces?

Agoraphobia. It also means having a sense of humiliation or hopelessness.

What antidepressant, which recently was approved for general anxiety disorder, inhibits the reuptake of NE and 5-HT?

Venlafaxine. (It also has a mild dopaminergic effect.)

What judgment states that the decision, by rights of autonomy and privacy, belongs to the patient, *but* if the patient is incompetent to decide,, the medical decision is based on subjective wishes?

Substituted judgment. It is made by the person who best knows the patient, not the closest relative.

What ethnic group has the highest adolescent suicide rate?

Native Americans

What are the three *microscopic* pathologic changes seen in Alzheimer's disease?

Senile plaques, neurofibrillary tangles, and granulovascular changes in neurons

When does most REM sleep occur, in the first or second half of sleep?

REM sleep occurs more often in the second half of sleep. The amount of REM sleep increases as the night goes on.

What is the name of the benzodiazepine *antagonist* used in the treatment of an overdose?

Flumazenil

What type of test asks a patient to draw a scene, attempting to find out the individual's unconscious perceptions in his or her life?

Projective drawing. The artistic form is irrelevant, but the size, placement, erasures, and distortions are relevant.

What is the biochemical trigger for REM sleep?

Increased ACh to decreased NE levels. (NE pathway begins in the pons and regulates REM sleep.)

What neuropsychologic test shows nine designs to the patient, then asks for recall of as many as possible?

Bender Visual Motor Gestalt Test

What are the three characteristics of ADHD?

1. Short attention span
2. Impulsivity
3. Hyperactivity

Is suicidal ideation a component of *normal* grief?

It is **rare** with normal grief; however, it is relatively common in depression

In what stage of sleep is it *easiest* to arouse a sleeping individual?

During REM sleep

What scale separates things into groups without defining the relationship between them?

Nominal scale (categorical, e.g., male or female)

What specifies how accurately the *sample values* and the *true values* of the population lie within a given range?

Confidence interval. It is a way of admitting estimation for the population.

If the family member of a patient asked you to withhold information, would you?

For the USMLE Step 1 the answer is no, but if the information would do more harm than good, withhold. This is very rare but it does occur.

What AD dementia has a defect in *chromosome 4*, onset between the ages of 30 and 40, choreoathetosis, and progressive deterioration to an infantile state?

Huntington's chorea. (Death in 15–20 years, often via suicide.)

What percentage of children born to HIV-positive mothers will test positive for HIV at *birth*?

100%, with about 20% remaining positive after 1 year

Name the reaction that appears in babies who are temporarily deprived of their usual caretaker. (This reaction usually begins around 6 months of age, peaks around 8 months, and decreases at 12 months.)

Separation anxiety

Which drug is used to treat opioid withdrawal, ADHD, and sometimes Tourette's syndrome?

Clonidine

What chromosome is autism linked to?

Chromosome 15

What type of correlation is defined as

    Two variables that go together in the *same direction*?

Positive correlation

    Two variables with *no linear relation* to one another?

Zero correlation

    One variable that diminishes in the presence of the other?

Negative correlation

When the results of a test are compared to findings for a *normative* group, what form of reference does the objective test use?

Norm reference (i.e., 75% of the students in the class will pass)

What hypothesis states that the findings of a test are a *result of chance*?

Null hypothesis (what you hope to disprove)

What is the term to describe the inability to feel any pleasant emotions?

Anhedonia

What is the term for involuntary constriction of the outer third of the vagina to prevent penile penetration?

Vaginismus; it is the female counterpart of premature ejaculation.

What is the term for the same results achieved again on testing a subject a second or third time?

Test–retest reliability

At what age does a child develop

> **Endogenous smile?**   At birth (reflex)

> **Exogenous smile?**   8 weeks (response to a face)

> **Preferential smile?**   12 to 16 weeks (in response to mother's face)

Per Freud, with what part of the unconscious are sex and aggression (instincts) associated?   Id

What enzyme is inhibited by disulfiram?   Aldehyde dehydrogenase. When this enzyme is blocked, acetaldehyde builds up, and its presence in excess results in nausea and hypotension.

What type of questions should you begin with when a patient seeks your medical opinion?   It is best to begin with open-ended questions, allowing patients to describe in their own words what troubles them. You can then move to closed-ended questions when narrowing the diagnosis.

What type of scheduled reinforcement states that after a desired response, the reinforcement is given

> **On a *set time* schedule?**   Fixed interval

> **After a *set number* of responses?**   Fixed ratio (rewards set behaviors)

> **Varying in *time*?**   Variable interval

> **Varying in the *number of responses*?**   Variable ratio
> If it is based on time, it is an *interval*, and if it is based on the number of responses, it is a *ratio*.

At what stage of psychosexual development (according to Freud) do children fear castration?	Phallic stage (4–6 years)

What is the label given to an individual whose IQ is

130	Very superior (<2.5% of the population)
110 to 119	High average
80 to 89	Low average
70 to 79	Borderline
90 to 109	Average
Below 69	Mentally disabled
120 to 129	Superior

At what stage of sleep is hCG output elevated?	Stage 4

Can incidence, prevalence, and cause and effect be assessed in

Case control studies?	Case control studies cannot assess incidence or prevalence, but they can determine causal relationships.
Cross-sectional studies?	Cross-sectional studies determine prevalence, not incidence or cause and effect.
Cohort studies?	Cohort studies determine incidence and causality, not prevalence.
Can a physician *commit* a patient?	NO!! Remember, only a judge can commit a patient. A physician can detain a patient (maximum is for 48 hours).

What are the five pieces of information considered necessary for fully informed consent?

1. Benefits of the procedure
2. Purpose of the procedure
3. Risks of the procedure
4. The nature of the procedure (what you are doing)
5. The alternative to this procedure and its availability

(Don't forget the last one; this is where physicians get in trouble.)

What is the term for the number of individuals who have an attribute or disease at a *particular point in time*?

Prevalence rate

What is the term for the degree to which a test measures what it is intended to measure?

Validity (remember, reliability is necessary but not the only thing needed for validity)

What Freudian psyche component is described as

The urges, sex aggression, and "primitive" processes?

Id (pleasure principle)

The conscience, morals, beliefs (middle of the road)?

Superego

Reality, rationality, language basis?

Ego

What medication is used to help alcoholics avoid relapse by decreasing *glutamate receptor activity*?

Acamprosate (the number of glutamate receptors increases with chronic alcohol abuse)

What is the term for new made-up words?

Neologisms. Thomas Jefferson noted, "Necessity obliges us to neologize." (Abnormal use of neologisms is known as neolalism.)

What rate removes any difference between two populations, based on a variable, to makes groups equal?

Standardized rate

Can *committed* mentally ill patients refuse medical treatment?

Yes. The only civil liberty they lose is the freedom to come and go as they please.

What is the term for any stimulus that *increases* the probability of a response happening?

Reinforcement

Does REM deprivation interfere with performance on *simple* tasks?

No, but it does interfere with performing complex tasks and decreases attention to detail. (Be careful post call!)

Name the *cluster C* personality disorder:

   Gets others to assume responsibility, is subordinate, and is fearful of being alone and caring for self

Dependent

   Orderly, inflexible, perfectionist; makes rules, lists, order; doesn't like change, has a poor sense of humor, and needs to keep a routine

Obsessive-compulsive

   Sensitive to criticism, shy, anxious; socially isolated but yearns to be in the crowd

Avoidant

What is the term for a complete aversion to all sexual contact?

Sexual aversion disorder

What type of symptoms in schizophrenia are associated with

Dopamine receptors?

Type I symptoms (positive); schizophrenics have them, but otherwise healthy persons do not.

Muscarinic receptors (ACh)?

Type II symptoms (negative); otherwise healthy persons have them, but schizophrenics do not.

What general pattern of sleep is described by slowing of EEG rhythms (high voltage and slower synchronization), muscle contractions, and lack of eye movement or mental activity?

NREM sleep. Remember awake body, sleeping brain

Is spousal abuse a *mandatory* reportable offense?

No, it is not a mandatory reportable offense (if you can believe it). Child and elderly abuse are mandatory reportable offenses.

What is the key issue surrounding teenagers' maturation?

Formation of an identity through issues of independence and rebellion; they define who they are.

What is the relationship between *chance of error* and

Standard deviation?

As the standard deviation increases, the greater the chance of error.

Sample size?

As sample size increases, the lower the chance of error.

Name the *cluster B* personality disorder:

Colorful, dramatic, extroverted, seductive, and unable to hold long-term relationships	Histrionic
In a constant state of crisis, promiscuous, unable to tolerate anxiety-causing situations, afraid of being alone, and having intense but brief relationships	Borderline
Criminal behavior; lacking friends, reckless, and unable to conform to social norms	Antisocial
Grandiose sense of self-importance; demands constant attention; fragile self-esteem; can be charismatic	Narcissistic
In what organ system would you attempt to localize a sign for shaken baby syndrome"? What do you look for?	Look for broken blood vessels in the baby's eyes.
What case is known as "let nature take its course"?	Infant Doe. Generally, parents cannot forego lifesaving treatment, but this case states that there are exceptions to the rule.
If the *P* value is less than or equal to .05, what do you do to the null hypothesis?	Reject it
What disorder is characterized by an alternating pattern of depressed mood with periods of hypomania for more than 2 years?	Cyclothymia (nonpsychotic bipolar). Patients are ego syntonic.

What projective test asks the patient to tell a story about what is going on in the pictures, evaluating the conflicts, drives, and emotions of the individual?

TAT

What has proved to be the best way to extinguish enuresis?

Bell pad

What scale assesses a *rank order* classification but *does not* tell the difference between the two groups?

Ordinal scale (e.g., faster/slower, taller/shorter)

What is associated with prolonged lithium use?

Hypothyroidism. (TSH levels must be monitored.)

What scale has a *true zero point*, graded into equal increments, and also orders them?

Ratio scale

By what age should children be able to draw the following figures?

   Triangle

6 years old

   Cross

4 years old

   Diamond

7 years old

   Square

5 years old

   Circle

3 years old

   Rectangle

4.5 years old
(Alphabetic order except with a
    diamond last: circle, cross,
    rectangle, square, triangle)

What personality disorder affects 75% of the prison population?

Antisocial personality

What is the first formal IQ test used today for children aged 2 to 18?

Stanford-Binet Scale, developed in 1905, is useful in the very bright, the impaired, and children less than 6 years old.

What type of foods should patients taking MAOIs avoid? Why?

Foods rich in tyramine (e.g., cheese, dried fish, sauerkraut, chocolate, avocados, and red wine) should be avoided. Hypertensive crisis occurs when tyramine and MAOIs are mixed.

What form of anxiety, appearing at 6 months, peaking at 8 months, and disappearing by 1 year of age, is seen in the presence of unfamiliar people?

Stranger anxiety

What are the three stages that children aged 7 months to 5 years go through when they are separated from a primary caregiver for a long time?

1. Protest
2. Despair
3. Detachment

What five things are checked in the APGAR test?

1. Skin color
2. Heart rate
3. Reflexes
4. Muscle tone
5. Respiratory rate

APGAR, **A**ppearance, **P**ulse, **G**rimace, **A**ctivity, **R**espiration

What are the top three causes of infant mortality?

Birth defects, low birth weight (<1500 g) with NRDS, and SIDS

Do newborns have a preference for still or moving objects?

Moving objects, along with large bright objects with curves and complex designs.

What is the name of the 12-step program believed to be the most successful for the treatment of alcohol abuse?

Alcoholics Anonymous

How can you differentiate between a medial temporal lobe and a hippocampal lesion based on memory impairment?

Long-term memory is impaired in *hippocampal* lesions; it is spared in *medial temporal lobe* lesions.

What α_1-receptor blocker's major sexual side effect is priapism?

Trazodone

What is the central issue regarding the *Roe vs. Wade* decision (legalization of abortion)?

The *patient* decides about the health care she does or does not get even if it harms the fetus. This also means she can refuse blood transfusions even if it harms the fetus.

What part of the ANS is affected in the biofeedback model of *operant* conditioning?

The biofeedback model is based on the parasympathetic nervous system.

The proportion of *truly diseased* persons in the screened population who are *identified as diseased* refers to?

Sensitivity (it deals with the sick)

How far below ideal body weight are patients with anorexia nervosa?

At least 15%

True or false? According to social learning theory, people who believe that luck, chance, or the actions of others control their fate have an *internal* locus of control.

False. These beliefs are characteristic of people with an *external* locus of control.

What is the term for an inhibited female orgasm?

Anorgasmia. (The overall prevalence is 30%.)

What are the four exceptions to requirements for informed consent?

1. Incompetent patient (determined by the courts)
2. Therapeutic privilege (in the best interest of the patient when he or she is unable to answer)
3. Waiver signed by the patient
4. Emergency

What is the term for recurrent and persistent pain before, after, or during sexual intercourse?

Dyspareunia. It is a common complaint in women who have been raped or sexually abused.

What type of bias is it when the sample population is *not a true representative* of the population?

Selection bias

In what stage of sleep is it *hardest* to arouse a sleeping individual?

During stage 3 and 4 (remember, it is called deep sleep.)

What is the period between falling asleep and REM sleep called?

REM latency; normally it is about 90 minutes.

What case is best known for use of the "best interest standard"?

Brother Fox (Eichner vs. Dillon). The substituted standard could not apply because the patient had *never* been competent, so no one knew what the patient *would* have wanted. Therefore, the decision was based on what a "reasonable" person *would* have wanted.

What drug is used to prevent alcohol consumption by blocking aldehyde dehydrogenase?

Disulfiram

According to Freud, what facet of the psyche represents the internalized ideals and values of one's parents?

Superego

What pineal hormone's release is *inhibited* by daylight and *increased* dramatically during sleep?

Melatonin. It is a light-sensitive hormone that is associated with sleepiness.

What somatoform disorder is described as

Having a F:M ratio of 20:1, onset before age 30, and having 4 pains (2 gastrointestinal, 1 sexual, 1 neurologic)?

Somatization disorder

La belle indifférence, suggestive of true physical ailment because of alteration of function?

Conversion disorder

Unrealistic negative opinion of personal appearance, seeing self as ugly?

Body dysmorphic disorder

Preoccupied with illness or death, persisting despite reassurance, lasting longer than 6 months?

Hypochondriasis (they will begin with "I think I have . . .")

Severe, prolonged pain that persists with no cause being found, disrupts activities of daily living?

Somatoform pain disorder

What statistical test compares the means of *many groups* (>2) of a *single nominal variable* by using an interval variable?

One-way ANOVA

What disease is described by the following characteristics: multiple motor *and* vocal tics, average age of onset 7, a M:F ratio of 3:1, and association with *increased* levels of dopamine?

Tourette's syndrome; it is usually first reported by teachers as ADHD with symptoms of obsessive-compulsive disorder and learning disabilities.

In Parkinson's disease, what area of the basal ganglia has a *decreased* amount of dopamine?

Substantia nigra

What naturally occurring substances mimic the effects of opioids?

Enkephalins

What disorder, experienced more than half of the time for a 6-month period, is described as being fearful, worrisome, or impatient and having sleep disturbances, poor concentration, hyperactivity, and an overall sense of autonomic hyperactivity?

Generalized anxiety disorder

What percent of sexual abuse cases are committed by family members?

50%. The uncles and older siblings are the most likely perpetrators, although stepfathers also have a high rate.

***Kaiser-Fleischer* rings, abnormal copper metabolism, and *ceruloplasmin* deficiency characterize what disease, which may include symptoms of dementia when severe?**

Wilson's disease (Remember chromosome 13 and hepatolenticular degeneration)

To what does failure to resolve separation anxiety lead?

School phobia

What is the term to describe the *average*?

Mean

How does L-tryptophan affect sleep?

It increases REM and total sleep time.

Should information flow *from* the patient *to* the family or vice versa?

Your duty is to tell the patient, not the family. The patient decides who gets to know and who doesn't, not you.

Can parents withhold treatment from their children?

Yes, as long the illness does not threaten limb or life. If illness is critical or an emergency, treat the child.

What is the name of the hypothesis you are trying to *prove*?

Alternative hypothesis (what is left after the null has been defined)

What percent of unwed mothers are teenagers?

50%, with 50% of them having the child

What happens to REM, REM latency, and stage 4 sleep during major depression?

Increased REM sleep, decreased REM latency, and decreased stage 4 sleep, leading to early morning awakening

What 11–amino acid peptide is the neurotransmitter of sensory neurons that conveys *pain* from the periphery to the spinal cord?

Substance P. (Opioids relieve pain in part by blocking substance P.)

True or false? In a positively skewed curve the *mean* is greater than the *mode*.

False. In positively skewed distributions the mode is greater than the median is greater than the mean.(Remember to name a skewed distribution: the tail points in the direction of its name. Positive skew tails point to the positive end of a scale.)

What is the term to describe jumping from one topic to the next without any connection?

Loose association

What is the leading cause of school dropout?

Pregnancy

Name the four components of the narcoleptic tetrad.

1. Sleep paralysis
2. Hypnagogic hallucinations (while falling asleep)
3. Sleep attacks with excessive daytime sleepiness
4. Cataplexy (pathognomonic)
Narcolepsy is a disorder of REM sleep, with REM occurring within 10 minutes of sleep.

What happens to cortisol levels in sleep-deprived individuals?

Cortisol levels increase. Lymphocyte levels decrease in sleep-deprived individuals.

What is the period between going to bed and falling asleep called?

Sleep latency

What disorder is characterized by a depressed mood and a loss of interest or pleasure for more than 2 years?

Dysthymia, which is also known as nonpsychotic depression. (Think of it as the car running but not well.)

What form of conditioning is defined as a *new response* to an *old stimulus* resulting in a consequence?

Operant conditioning (reinforcement is after a response)

What pituitary hormone is *inhibited* during sleep?

TSH. 5-HT and prolactin increase during sleep, and dopamine levels decrease during sleep.

Based on *operant* conditioning, what type of reinforcement is described when

**   *Adding* a stimulus *stops* a behavior?**

Punishment

**   *Removing* a stimulus *stops* a behavior?**

Extinction

**   *Adding* a stimulus *reinforces* a behavior?**

Positive reinforcement

**   *Removing* a stimulus *reinforces* a behavior?**

Negative reinforcement

What is the formula to calculate IQ?

$(MA/CA) \times 100 = IQ$ score, where $MA =$ mental age and $CA =$ chronological age

What happens to NE levels in

**   Major depression?**

Decrease (5-HT and dopamine levels do the same)

**   Bipolar disorder?**

Increase (5-HT and dopamine levels do the same)

What law was adopted to shield physicians from liability when helping at the scene of an accident?	Good Samaritan Law. (Physicians are not required to stop and help.)
What is the term for the number of *new* events occurring in a population divided by the population *at risk*?	Incidence rate
What is the term to describe inability to recall the past and possible assumption of a completely new identity?	Dissociative fugue. (Patients are unaware of memory loss.)

What *classical* conditioning therapy or modification is described as

Pairing *noxious stimuli* to an inappropriate behavior?	Aversive conditioning
Forcing patients to *confront their fears* by being exposed to them until they are extinguished?	Exposure
Triage of a hierarchy of fears (from least to most), then teaching muscle relaxation techniques in the presence of those fears until the subject is not afraid anymore?	Systematic desensitization
Failure to accurately recall the past leads to what form of bias?	Recall bias. These problems arise in retrospective studies.

Regarding neuroleptics, what is the relationship between *potency* and *anticholinergic side effects*?

Inversely proportional: the higher the potency, the lower the anticholinergic side effects.

What potentially lethal side effect of clozapine should be monitored with frequent blood drawing?

Agranulocytosis; approximately 2% develop this side effect.

True or false? Being college educated increases a man's risk of having premature ejaculation.

True; also, stressful marriage, early sexual experiences in the back of a car, and sex with a prostitute all increase the risk of premature ejaculation.

What is the term for the rate measured for a *subgroup of a population*?

Specific rate (e.g., men aged 55–60)

In what stage of psychosexual development, according to Freud, do children resolve the Oedipus complex?

Latency stage (6–12 years)

Where is lithium metabolized and excreted?

95% in the kidneys; that's why adequate Na⁺ and fluid intake is essential.

At what age do children begin to understand the irreversibility of death?

At 8 to 9 years of age. Prior to this age they view death as a form of punishment.

What are the three benzodiazepines that do *not* undergo microsomal oxidation?

Oxazepam, temazepam, and lorazepam (OTL) (mnemonic: **O**utside **T**he **L**iver). They undergo glucuronide conjugation, not via the cytochrome p450 system.

What neuropsychologic test has five basic scales testing for the presence and localization of brain dysfunction?

The Halsted-Reitan battery. It consists of finger oscillation, speech sound perception, rhythm, tactual, and category testing.

What subtype of schizophrenia is characterized by

Childlike behaviors, unorganized speech and behaviors, poor grooming, incongruous smiling and laughter, and the worst prognosis?

Disorganized schizophrenia

***Stuporous* mute echopraxia and automatic obedience, *waxy* flexibility with rigidity of posture?**

Catatonic schizophrenia

Delusions of persecution and/or grandeur, auditory hallucinations, late onset, and the best prognosis?

Paranoid schizophrenia

If a patient cannot pay, can you refuse services?

No, you never refuse to treat a patient simply because he or she can't pay. You are a patient advocate.

Does alcoholism increase the rate of suicide?

Yes. It increases the rate of suicide to nearly 50 times that of the general population.

What is the term for the dementia characterized by decremental or patchy deterioration in cognitive function due to a cerebrovascular accident?

Vascular dementia. It is characterized as a stepwise deterioration in cognitive function.

What is the term for the difference between the highest and the lowest score in a population?

Range

How is sleep affected in a person with alcohol intoxication?

Decreased REM sleep and REM rebound during withdrawal

How many attacks are needed over _how much time_ before panic disorder is diagnosed?

Need 3 panic attacks over 3 weeks (remember, they come out of the blue.)

What axis I disorder is characterized by pronoun reversal, preference for inanimate objects, obliviousness to the external environment, lack of separation anxiety, and abnormalities in language development?

Autism. Head-banging, rocking, and self-injurious behaviors are also common in autism.

What major side effect of neuroleptics is characterized by pill rolling, shuffling gait, and tremors that abate during sleep?

Tardive dyskinesia. It persists even after treatment is discontinued and has no treatment. Focus is on monitoring for side effects and prevention.

If you report a suspected case of child abuse and are wrong, are you protected from legal liability?

Yes. This is done to help prevent underreporting out of fear of lawsuit. Remember that it is your duty to protect the child first, not worry about legal responsibility.

Can advance directives be _oral_?

Yes

Increased self-esteem, flight of ideas, decreased sleep, increased libido, weight loss, and erratic behavior are all symptoms of what disorder?

Bipolar disorder (manic-depressive disorder)

Is marital satisfaction higher for couples with or without children?	Without children (but don't think about this one for too long)
At what age does IQ stabilize?	From age 5 onward IQ stabilizes.

Name the *aphasia* based on these characteristics:

Nonfluent speech, telegraphic and ungrammatical; lesion in Brodmann's area 44; unimpaired comprehension	Broca's aphasia
Lesion in the *prefrontal* cortex; inability to speak spontaneously; unimpaired ability to repeat	Transcortical aphasia
Lesion is in the *parietal lobe* or *arcuate fibers* because the connection between Broca's and Wernicke's area is severed; word comprehension preserved; *inability* to write or speak the statement (can't tell you what you said)	Conduction aphasia
***Both* Broca's and Wernicke's areas damaged by lesion in the *presylvian speech area;* trouble repeating statements; poor comprehension with *telegraphic* speech**	Global aphasia

Lesion in Brodmann area 22; impaired comprehension; incoherent rapid, fluent speech; verbal paraphrasias; trouble repeating statements	Wernicke's aphasia
What rare form of dementia is associated with personality changes and affects the frontal and temporal lobes?	Pick's disease
Which drug is used to treat respiratory depression associated with an overdose of opioids?	Naloxone or naltrexone
What rate is indicated by 1 − specificity?	False-positive rate
When does most of the NREM sleep (stage 3 and 4) occur, in the first or second half of sleep?	The deepest sleep levels (stage 3 and 4) occur mostly in the first half of sleep.

Name the stages of sleep with these EEG patterns:

Disappearance of alpha waves, appearance of theta waves	Stage 1
Delta waves	Stage 3 and 4
Sawtooth waves, random low voltage pattern	REM
Alpha waves	Being awake
Sleep spindles, K-complexes	Stage 2

What is the drug of choice for treating ADHD?

Methylphenidate (Ritalin)

True or false? Prolactin levels can serve as a rough indicator of overall *dopamine* activity.

True. PIF is dopamine in the tuberoinfundibular system.

What is the term for failure to give up infantile patterns of behavior for mature ones?

Fixation (arrested development)

Is masturbation considered an *abnormal* sexual practice?

No. It is abnormal only if it interferes with normal sexual or occupational function.

Which benzodiazepine has the *longest* half-life?

Flurazepam

In the *classical conditioning* model, when a behavior is learned, what must occur to break the probability that a response will happen?

Stimulus generalization must stop. (Pairing of the unconditioned stimulus and the conditioned stimulus must cease.)

What is the most abundant neuron in the cerebellum?

The granule cell. Its neurotransmitter is glutamic acid, which is also the principal neurotransmitter of the visual pathways.

Name these *anxiety* defense mechanisms:

Separating oneself from the experience. The facts are accepted but the form is changed for protection.

Dissociation

Use of explanations to justify unacceptable behaviors.

Rationalization

Outburst to cover up true feelings (emotion is covered, not redirected).	Acting out
Use of an outlet for emotions (stuff flows downhill).	Displacement
Fact without feeling (la belle indifférence)	Isolation of affect
Replacing normal affect with "brain power"	Intellectualization
Unconsciously forgetting (forgetting that you forgot something!)	Repression
Fixing impulses by acting out the opposite of an unacceptable behavior	Undoing
Setting up to be let down (it is unconscious; if conscious, you're just rude)	Passive-aggressive
A complete opposite expression of your inward feeling (e.g., arguing all the time with someone you are attracted to when your feelings are not known)	Reaction formation

Name these *cluster A* personality disorders:

Odd, strange; has magical thinking; socially isolated, paranoid, lacks close friends; has incongruous affect	Schizotypal

Socially withdrawn, seen as eccentric but happy to be alone	Schizoid
Baseline mistrust; carries grudges; afraid to open up; uses projection as defense mechanism; lacks hallucinations or delusions	Paranoid

What statistical method do you use when analyzing

Cross-sectional studies?	Chi-square.
Cohort studies?	Relative risk and/or attributable risk. (*Cohort* studies deal with incidence.)
Case control studies?	Odds ratio. (*Case control studies* deal with prevalence.)

If a patient asks you a question and you do not know the answer, do you tell a white lie or simply not respond?	Absolutely not! Answer any question you are asked.
True or false? There is a strong *positive* correlation between IQ and academic achievement.	True. IQ correlates well with education and academic achievement but is not a predictor of success.
What is the term for headaches, inability to concentrate, sleep disturbances; avoidance of associated stimuli; reliving events as dreams or flashbacks following a psychologically stressful event *beyond the normal range of expectation*?	Posttraumatic stress disorder. (Important: symptoms must be exhibited for longer than 1 month.)

What is the term for a schizophrenic episode lasting longer than 30 days with full return to former functioning capacity?

Brief psychotic disorder. (In schizophreniform disorder the symptoms last longer than 6 months.)

What is the primary method of nonverbal communication of emotional states?

Facial expression (the second is vocal intonation)

What type of mortality rate is defined as the number of deaths

In the population?

Crude mortality rate

From a specific cause *per population*?

Cause-specific mortality rate

From a specific cause *per all deaths*?

Proportionate mortality rate

From a specific cause *per number of persons with the disease*?

Case fatality rate

Does being a female physician increase or decrease the risk of suicide?

Being a female physician increases the risk of suicide nearly four times the general population.

Are sexually abused females more likely to have learning disabilities than the general population?

Yes, by three to four times. Having multiple sexual partners, being overweight, and pelvic pain and/or inflammatory disorders are also likely to be seen in sexually abused females.

What form of bias is due to false estimates of survival rates?

Lead-time bias (remember, patients don't live longer with the disease; they are diagnosed sooner.)

The probability that a person with *a positive test result is truly positive* refers to what value?

Positive predictive value

Objective tests that base the result of the examination on a *preset standard* use what form of reference?

Criterion-referenced tests. You need a certain number correct to pass (e.g., the USMLE).

True or false? A patient can refuse a feeding tube.

True. It is considered medical treatment, so it can be withdrawn or refused. (Remember the Cruzan case.)

What are the CAGE questions?

Cut down (ever tried and failed?)
Annoyed (criticism makes angry?)
Guilty (about drinking behavior?)
Eye opener (drinking to shake out the cobwebs?)

What type of scale is graded into equal increments, showing not only any difference but how much?

Interval scale (a ruler, for example)

With what stage of sleep are bruxisms associated?

Teeth grinding is associated with stage 2 sleep.

What rate is indicated by 1 − sensitivity?

False-negative rate

What drug is being given to HIV-positive mothers during labor and to the children after birth to decrease the risk of mother-to-child HIV transmission?

Nevirapine; it cuts the rate from 20% to 10%. AZT is also used, cutting the rate from 20% to 10%.

What is the name of depression and mania alternating within a 48- to 72-hour period?

Rapid cycling bipolar disorder

Aroused EEG pattern (fast low voltage and desynchronization), *saccadic* eye movements, ability to dream, and sexual arousal are all associated with what general pattern of sleep?

REM sleep. Remember, awake brain in a sleeping body.

What is the *teratogenic* effect associated with lithium?

Epstein-cardiac anomaly of the tricuspid valve

What is the triad of NPH?

Dementia
Urinary incontinence
Gait apraxia
(NPH = wet, wacky, wobbly)

True or false? Only men have refractory sexual periods.

Sad but true. Some women can have multiple successive orgasms.

In which syndrome does a person present with intentionally produced physical ailments with the intent to assume the sick role?

Münchhausen's syndrome (factitious disorder)

Name these *mature* defense mechanisms:

Preparing for an upcoming event

Anticipation

Helping others without expecting any return

Altruism

Converting an unacceptable impulse to a socially acceptable form (Hint: it is the most mature of all defense mechanisms)

Sublimation

Forgetting on purpose (so you can actually remember it)	Suppression
Easing anxiety with laughter	Humor

Name the area of the cerebral cortex with the function described:

Speech; critical for *personality*, concentration, initiating and stopping tasks (do one thing and begin a new without completion of the first), abstract thought, and memory and higher-order mental functions	Frontal lobe
Language, memory, and emotion (Hint: *herpesvirus* infects here commonly)	Temporal lobe
Intellectual processing of *sensory* information, with the *left* (dominant) processing verbal information, the *right* processing visual-spatial orientation	Parietal lobe
Initiation and control of movements	Basal ganglia
Skill-based memory, verbal recall, *balance*, refined voluntary movements	Cerebellum
Important for REM sleep; origin of NE pathway	Pons

Motivation, memory, *emotions*, violent behaviors, sociosexual behaviors, conditioned responses

Limbic system

Recall of objects, distances, and scenes; *visual* input processed here

Occipital lobe

What is the degree to which two measures are related? Does it imply causation?

Correlation. No, correlation does not imply causation.

What is the most common form of dementia?

Alzheimer's (dementia of Alzheimer's type, DAT). (Remember, Alzheimer's constitutes 65% of dementias seen in patients 65 years old.)

What is the *only* drug that does *not* have an intoxication?

Nicotine (but it sure has a nasty withdrawal!)

What is the term to describe homosexuals who

Are *comfortable* with their own person and *agree* with their sense of self?

Ego syntonic

Are *uncomfortable* with their own person and *disagree* with their sense of self?

Ego dystonic

Which benzodiazepine has the *shortest* half-life?

Triazolam

What statistical test compares the means of *groups* generated by *two nominal variables* by using an interval variable?

Two-way ANOVA. It allows the test to check several variables at the same time.

What are the two ways to leave the prevalence pot?

Recovery and death

What aspects of sleep are affected during benzodiazepine use?

REM and stage 4 sleep; they decrease.

What is the term to describe a man who has

Never been able to achieve an erection?

Primary erectile disorder

The ability to have an erection sometimes and other times not?

Selective erectile disorder

Used to be able to achieve an erection but now cannot?

Secondary erectile disorder
(Male erectile disorder is the same as impotence.)

What stage of sleep is associated with somnambulism?

Sleepwalking is associated with stage 4 and occurs most often in the first third of sleep.

What are the three surrogate criteria?

1. What did the patient want?
2. What would the patient say?
3. What is in the patient's best interests?

True or false? Four-fifths of those who attempt suicide first give a warning.

True; 80% have visited a doctor in the previous 6 months. And 50% within the last month!

Can a patient refuse life-saving treatment for religious reasons?

Yes. (Remember, Jehovah's witnesses refuse blood transfusions.)

What form of bias occurs when the experimenter's expectation inadvertently is expressed to the subjects, producing the desired effects? How can it be eliminated?

Pygmalion effect (experimenter expectancy). This can be eliminated with double-blind studies.

What type of hallucination occurs during *awakening*?

Hypnopompic hallucinations occur during awakening, whereas hypnagogic hallucinations occur while one is falling asleep.

When attempting to make up sleep, what stage of sleep is recovered?

About 80% of stage 4 sleep is recovered, approximately half of REM is recovered, and only one-third of total sleep is ever made up.

What is backward masking, and is there a positive correlation with schizophrenic patients?

When showing two pictures in rapid succession, you split the pictures half a second apart, resulting in the second picture *masking* the first (indicating poor short-term memory). This is seen in nearly 33% of schizophrenic patients.

True or false? Being single increases your risk of suicide.

False. Separation, divorce, being widowed, and unemployment increase your risk, but being single does not.

True or false? Serious psychiatric illness is more common after abortion than childbirth.

False. Childbirth carries five times as much risk of serious psychiatric illness as abortion.

What type of error is made if you *accept* the null hypothesis when it is *false*?

Type II error (beta error). (Remember it as saying something doesn't work when it does.)

Most sleep time is spent in what stage of sleep?

Stage 2, which accounts for approximately 45% of total sleep time, with REM occupying 20%.

In a negatively skewed curve is the *mean* greater than the *mode*?

Yes. In a negatively skewed distribution the mean is greater than the median is greater than the mode.

What axis I disorder is characterized by a clinically significant syndrome that affects

Adjustment disorder. It is a diagnosis of exclusion (used if no other choice).

social, occupational, and/or academic achievement; occurs less than 3 months *after* a stressor; and abates less than 6 months *after* the stressor is removed?

What type of personality test is the Rorschach inkblot test, objective or projective?

Projective test. Most tests with a wide range of possibilities for the answers are projective.

What statistical test checks to see whether the groups are different by comparing the means of *two groups* from a *single nominal variable*?

The T-test (used when comparing two groups)

What antipsychotic movement disorder can occur at any time and is characterized by a subjective sense of discomfort that brings on restlessness, pacing, sitting down, and getting up?

Akathisia

What form of depression is due to abnormal metabolism of melatonin?

Seasonal affective disorder (treat with bright light therapy)

What three circumstances allow a child to be committed to institutional care?

1. The child poses an imminent danger to self or others.
2. The child is unable to self-care daily at the appropriate developmental level.
3. The parents or guardians have no control over the child or will not promise to ensure the child's safety even though they refuse hospitalization.

What *operant* conditioning therapy or modification is described as

Reinforcing successive attempts that lead to the desired goal (gradual improvement)?

Shaping (successive approximation)

Having a stimulus take over the control of the behavior (unintentionally)?

Stimulus control

Providing the person with information regarding his or her *internal* responses to stimuli with methods of controlling them?

Biofeedback

Removing a reinforcement (without the patient knowing) gradually over time to stop a condition?

Fading

Stopping the reinforcement that is leading to an undesired behavior?

Extinction

The DSM-IV-TR is scored on the basis of five axes of diagnosis. In what axis would you place

Psychosocial and environmental problems (stressors)?

Axis IV

Medical or physical ailments?

Axis III

Personality and mental disorders?	Axis II
Global assessment of function?	Axis V
Clinical disorders (e.g., schizophrenia)?	Axis I

Should you refer a patient to a form of folk medicine even if you don't believe in it?

Actually, yes. You should encourage your patient to try other forms of medicine as long as they are not contraindicated with the patient's preexisting illness. You must be able to accept the health beliefs of your patients, even if you don't agree.

In regard to motor development during infancy, choose the motor response that happens *first*.

Release or grasp	Grasp proceeds release
Proximal or distal progression	Proximal to distal progression
Radial or ulnar progression	Ulnar to radial progression
Palms up or down	Palms-up before palms-down maneuvers

What are the strongest determinants of gender identity?

Parental assignment and culture (not biology)

With what stage of sleep are night terrors associated?

NREM sleep. Night terrors are dreams that we are unable to recall.

What type of bias is it when the information is distorted because of the *way it is gathered*?

Measurement bias

What term describes senseless repetition of words or phrases?

Verbigeration

Who decides *competency* and *sanity*?

The courts. These are legal, not medical terms.

Name these *narcissistic* defense mechanisms:

Everything in the world is perceived as either *good* or *bad*. No middle ground; it is all extremes.

Splitting

Not allowing reality to penetrate because afraid of becoming aware of painful aspect of reality.

Denial

Person takes his or her own feelings, beliefs, wishes, and so on and thinks they are someone else's. (e.g., a cheating man thinks his wife is unfaithful)

Projection

Which is the conditioned response, the conditioned stimulus, the unconditioned response, the unconditioned stimulus in this case? A patient has blood withdrawn and faints. The next time she goes to have blood taken, she faints at the sight of the needle.

The blood withdrawn is the unconditioned stimulus, inducing the unconditioned response (fainting). The needle is part of the blood-drawing procedure and is the conditioned stimulus (unconditioned and conditioned stimuli are paired) resulting in the conditioned response (fainting at the sight of the needle).

What three actions should take place when one person threatens the life of another? (Hint: think of the Tarasoff decision.)

1. Notify police.
2. Try to detain the person making the threat.
3. Notify the threatened victim.

Name the area of the cerebral cortex affected by the description of the effects, symptoms, and results of the *lesion*.

Apathy, *aggression*, inability to learn new material, and memory problems	Limbic system
Apathy, *poor grooming*, poor ability to think abstractly, decreased drive, poor attention span (Hint: if the lesion is in the dominant hemisphere, the patient will develop Broca's aphasia)	Dorsal prefrontal cortex
Euphoria, delusions, thought disorders, Wernicke's aphasia, *auditory* hallucinations (Hint: the lesion is in the *left* hemisphere)	Dominant temporal lobe
Agraphia, acalculia, finger agnosia, right–left disorientation	Dominant parietal lobe (Gerstmann's syndrome)
Withdrawn, fearful, *explosive* moods, violent outbursts, and loss of inhibitions	Orbitomedial frontal lobe
Denial of illness, hemineglect, construction apraxia (can't arrange matchsticks)	Nondominant parietal lobe
Denies being *blind*, cortical *blindness*	Occipital lobe (Anton's syndrome if it is due to bilateral posterior cerebral artery occlusions)

Dysphoria, irritability, musical and visual abilities decreased	Nondominant temporal lobe
What hormone's release is strongly associated with stage 4 sleep?	GH. The largest output of GH in a 24-hour period is during stage 4 sleep.
What is the male-to-female ratio for *committing* suicide?	M:F 4:1 committing, but M:F ratio of attempts is 1:3 (males commit more but females try it more)
What is the term for the total percentage of correct answers selected on a screening test?	Accuracy (think of it as all the trues, because they are the ones correctly identified)
What type of error is made if you *reject* the null hypothesis when it is *true*?	Type I error (alpha error). (Remember it as saying something works when it doesn't.) The chance of a type I error occurring is the P value.
If one event precludes another event, their probabilities are combined by what method?	Addition (They are mutually exclusive.)
True or false? Marriage emancipates a child less than 17 years old.	True; military service and independent self-care by a child over 13 years old also emancipate.
What term describes the inability to recall personal information, commonly associated with trauma?	Amnesia. (The person is aware of the memory loss.)
What is the most stressful event as determined by the Holmes and Rahe scale?	The death of a spouse. The higher the score, the greater the risk of developing an illness in the next 6 months.
What renal side effect is commonly seen in patients taking lithium?	Nearly 25% of patients taking lithium develop polyuria and polydipsia.

What statistical test, using *nominal* data only, checks whether two variables are *independent events*?

Chi-square (when you are in doubt and have nominal data, use chi-square)

What is the term for repetitive actions blocking recurring bad thoughts?

Compulsions. They are actions done to fix the bad thoughts. Obsessions are the thoughts.

True or false? A patient has to *prove* his or her *competency*.

False. You need clear evidence the patient is not competent; if you are unsure, assume the patient is competent.

True or false? Panic attacks can be induced by hyperventilation or carbon dioxide.

True. Yohimbine, sodium lactate, and epinephrine can also induce panic attacks; they are considered *panicogens*.

In what study, for ethical reasons, is no group left out of intervention?

Crossover study

Shuffling gait, cogwheel rigidity, masklike facies, pill-rolling tremor, and bradykinesia describe what form of dementia?

Parkinson's disease

Anhedonia, lack of motivation, feelings of worthlessness, decreased sex drive, insomnia, and recurrent thoughts for at least 2 weeks, representing a change from previous level of function, describes what disorder?

Unipolar disorder (major depression)

What form of dementia is characterized by onset at age 40 to 50, rapid progression, infection by a *prion*, and death within 2 years?

Creutzfeldt-Jakob's disease. Patients first develop vague somatic complaints and anxiety, rapidly followed by dysarthria, myoclonus, ataxia, and choreoathetosis.

The most *frequent number* occurring in a population is what?	Mode
Movement disorders are associated with what dopamine pathway (what part of the brain)?	Nigrostriatal pathways (basal ganglia)
What neurotransmitter is associated with *sedation* and *weight gain*?	Histamine
The probability that a person with a *negative test result* is *truly disease free* refers to what value?	Negative predictive value
What are the five Kübler-Ross stages of death and dying? Must they be completed in order?	Denial Anger Bargaining Depression Acceptance No, they can be skipped, repeated, and completed out of sequence.
What *P* value defines whether the hull hypothesis should or should not be rejected?	$P = .05$; $P < .05$ rejects the null hypothesis
What hormone level increases in the first 3 hours of sleep?	Prolactin
What is the most widely used class of antidepressants?	SSRIs
What happens to prevalence as the number of long-term survivors increases?	Prevalence increases. (Remember, prevalence can decrease in only two ways, recovery and death.)

What is the primary predisposing factor for vascular dementia?	Hypertension

What *paraphilia* is defined as

Sexual urges toward children?	Pedophilia
Deriving sexual pleasure from watching others having sex, grooming, or undressing?	Voyeurism
Having a recurrent desire to expose the genitals to strangers?	Exhibitionism
Deriving sexual pleasure from other peoples' pain?	Sadism
Deriving sexual pleasure from being abused or in pain?	Masochism
Having sex with cadavers?	Necrophilia
Sexual fantasies or practices with animals?	Zoophilia
Combining sex with defecation?	Coprophilia
Combining sex with urination?	Urophilia
A male rubbing his genitals on a fully clothed female to achieve orgasm?	Frotteurism

Name the neurotransmitter at the *neuromuscular junctions* for all of the *voluntary muscles* in the body.

ACh; think about the ANS.

What are the pharmacologic effects seen sexually with

    α_1-Blockers?

Impaired ejaculation

    Serotonin?

Inhibited orgasm

    β-Blockers?

Impotence

    Trazodone?

Priapism

    Dopamine agonists?

Increased erection and libido

    Neuroleptics?

Erectile dysfunction

What is the term for the point on a scale that divides the population into *two equal parts*?

Median (think of it as the halfway point)

True or false? Pregnancy ensures emancipation.

False

True or false? Paranoid and catatonic schizophrenia are good prognostic predictors.

True. Being female, having positive symptoms, quick onset, and family history of *mood* disorders are all good prognostic predictors of schizophrenia.

What happens to prevalence as incidence increases?

Prevalence increases.

What type of correlation compares two *interval variables*?

Pearson correlation

What term is defined as a patient unconsciously placing his or her thoughts and feelings on the physician in a caregiver or parent role?

Transference. When it is from the physician to the patient it is called *countertransference*.

What phase of Food and Drug Administration approval tests

The efficacy and occurrence of side effects in large group of patient volunteers?

Phase III. It is considered the definitive test.

The safety in healthy volunteers?

Phase I

The protocol and dose levels in a small group of patient volunteers?

Phase II

In biostatistics, what are the three criteria required to increase power?

1. Large sample size
2. Large effect size
3. Type I error is greater

If the occurrence of one event had *nothing to do* with the occurrence of another event, how do you combine their probabilities?

Since they are independent events, their probabilities would be multiplied.

What type of random controlled test is least subjective to bias?

Double-blind study. It is the most scientifically rigorous study known.

Why isn't the incidence of a disease decreased when a new treatment is initiated?

Because incidence is defined as new events; treatment does not decrease the number of new events. It does decrease the number of individuals with the event (prevalence would decrease).

3 Biochemistry

What are the three posttranscriptional modifications?

1. 7-methyl guanine cap on the 5′ end
2. Addition of the poly(A) tail to the 3′ end
3. Removal of introns

What AA is the major carrier of nitrogen byproducts from most tissues in the body?

Glutamine

What two AAs have a pKa of 4?

Aspartic acid and glutamic acid

How many acetyl CoAs per glucose enter into the TCA cycle?

2 acetyl CoA per glucose, producing **12 ATPs per acetyl CoA,** resulting in a **total of 24 ATPs produced from glucose** (via acetyl CoA) enter the **TCA cycle**

What topoisomerase makes ssDNA cuts, requires no ATP, relaxes supercoils, and acts as the swivel in front of the replication fork?

Topoisomerase I (Relaxase)

In *prokaryotes*, what is the name of the RNA sequence that ribosomes bind to so translation can occur?

Shine-Dalgarno sequence

Name the pattern of genetic transmission: both M and F are affected; M-to-M transmission may

Autosomal recessive

be present; both parents must be carriers; the trait skips generations; two mutant alleles are needed for disease; and affected children may be born of unaffected adults?

What factors are needed for translation in prokaryotes?

Elongation factor-G and GTP

What three AAs must patients with maple syrup urine disease not eat?

Isoleucine, leucine, and valine

How many high-energy bonds are used to activate an AA?

2 ATPs, via the amino acyl tRNA synthase enzyme

What water-soluble vitamin deficiency results in *pellagra*?

Niacin (B_3)

What glycolytic enzyme has a high V_{max}, high K_m, and low affinity for glucose?

Glucokinase

How many ATPs are generated per acetyl coenzyme A (CoA)?

12 ATPs per acetyl CoA that enter the tricarboxylic acid (TCA) cycle (Krebs cycle)

What cytoplasmic pathway produces *NADPH* and is a source of *ribose 5-phosphate*?

HMP shunt

What is the main inhibitor of pyruvate dehydrogenase?

Acetyl CoA (pyruvate to acetyl CoA)

Where on the *codon* and *anticodon* does the wobble hypothesis take place?

3' end of the codon (third position) on **mRNA** and 5' end of the anticodon (first position) on **tRNA**.

What DNA excision and repair enzyme is deficient in patients with xeroderma pigmentosum?	Excision endonuclease, which removes thiamine dimers from DNA
What form of bilirubin is carried on albumin?	Unconjugated (indirect)
What are the two *ketogenic* AAs?	Leucine and lysine
Which organisms have polycistronic mRNA?	Prokaryotes. **P**olycistronic and **p**rokaryotes both start with **P**.
As what compound do the carbons for fatty acid synthesis leave the mitochondria?	Citrate, via the citrate shuttle
What four substances increase the rate of gluconeogenesis?	1. Glucagon 2. NADH 3. Acetyl CoA 4. ATP
With what three enzymes is TPP associated?	1. α-Ketoglutarate dehydrogenase 2. Pyruvate dehydrogenase 3. Transketolase
What test uses very small amounts of DNA that can be amplified and analyzed without the use of Southern blotting or cloning?	PCR
What apoprotein is required for the release of chylomicrons from the epithelial cells into the lymphatics?	apo B-48
What enzyme catalyzes the covalent bonding of the	**Aminoacyl-tRNA synthetase** uses 2 ATPs for this reaction.

AA's carboxyl group to the 3' end of tRNA?

What must be supplemented in patients with medium-chain acyl CoA dehydrogenase (MCAD) deficiency?

Short-chain fatty acids

What form of AA is found only in collagen?

Hydroxyproline

In a diabetic patient, to what does aldose reductase convert glucose?

Sorbitol (resulting in cataracts)

What enzyme catalyzes the rate-limiting step in cholesterol metabolism?

HMG-CoA reductase

What is the term for the pH at which the structure carries *no charge*?

pI (isoelectric point)

What enzyme catalyzes the rate-limiting step in gluconeogenesis?

Fructose-1,6-bisphosphatase

What is the drug of choice in treating a patient with hyperuricemia due to *underexcretion* of uric acid?

Probenecid, a uricosuric agent

What enzyme deficiency results in darkening of the urine when exposed to air?

Homogentisate oxidase deficiency is seen in patients with alcaptonuria.

In *eukaryotes*, what transcription factor binds to the TATA box before RNA polymerase II can bind?

Transcription factor IID

What enzyme produces an RNA primer in the 5′-3′ direction and is essential to DNA replication because DNA polymerases are unable to synthesize DNA without an RNA primer?	Primase
What enzyme catalyzes the rate-limiting step in fatty acid synthesis?	Acetyl CoA carboxylase
Name the *eukaryotic* DNA polymerase based on the following information:	
Replicates mitochondrial DNA	DNA polymerase-γ
Synthesizes the lagging strand during replication	DNA polymerase-α
Synthesizes the leading strand during replication	DNA polymerase-δ
What is the order of fuel use in a prolonged fast?	1. Glucose from liver glycogen 2. Glucose from gluconeogenesis 3. Body protein 4. Body fat
Which way will the O_2 dissociation curve shift with the addition of 2,3-bisphosphoglycerate (2,3-BPG) to adult hemoglobin (Hgb)?	Shifts it to the right
What enzyme of pyrimidine synthesis is inhibited by the following?	
5-FU	Thymidylate synthase
Methotrexate	Dihydrofolate reductase

Hydroxyurea	Ribonucleotide reductase
What is found in the R group if the AA is acidic? Basic?	If a **carboxyl** group is the R group, it is **acidic;** if an **amino** group is the R group, it is said to be **basic.**
What gluconeogenic *mitochondrial* enzyme requires biotin?	Pyruvate carboxylase
What factors are needed for translocation in eukaryotes?	EF-2 and GTP
DNA replication occurs during what phase of the cell cycle?	S phase
What is the end product of purine catabolism?	Uric acid
What causes transcription to stop in eukaryotes?	The poly(A) site on the DNA
What enzyme of the TCA cycle catalyzes the production of the following:	
FADH$_2$	Succinate dehydrogenase
GTP	Succinyl CoA synthetase
NADH (hint: 3 enzymes)	Isocitrate dehydrogenase, α-ketoglutarate dehydrogenase, and malate dehydrogenase
What form of alcohol causes blindness?	Methanol (wood alcohol)
How many base pairs upstream is the *prokaryotic* TATA box promoter?	There are two bacterial promoter regions upstream. The **TATA box is -10 base pairs** upstream, and the -35 promoter site is self-explanatory.

What are the two essential fatty acids?

Linoleic acid and linolenic acid

During a prolonged fast, why is the brain unable to use fatty acids?

Fatty acids **cannot** cross the blood-brain barrier; therefore, they **cannot** be used as an energy source.

What type of jaundice is seen in Rotor's syndrome?

Conjugated (direct) hyperbilirubinemia

If a sample of DNA has 30% T, what is the percent of C?

Solved as 30% T + 30% A = 60%; therefore, C + G = 40%; then **C = 20%** and G = 20% (example of Chargaff's rule)

From where is the energy for gluconeogenesis derived?

β-Oxidation of fatty acids

Name the type of mutation:

The deletion or addition of a *base*

Frameshift

New codon specifies a *different* AA

Missense

Unequal crossover in *meiosis* with loss of protein function

Large segment deletions

New codon specifies for the *same* AA

Silent

New codon specifies for a *stop* codon

Nonsense

What form of bilirubin can cross the blood-brain barrier?

Unconjugated free bilirubin

What AA is broken down into N_2O, causing an increase in cyclic guanosine

Arginine

monophosphate (cGMP) of smooth muscle, hence vasodilation?

What is needed to produce a double bond in a fatty acid chain in the endoplasmic reticulum?	NADPH, O_2, and cytochrome b_5
What are the vitamin K–dependent coagulation factors?	Factors II, VII, IX, X, and proteins C and S
Is the hydroxyl (−OH) end of DNA and RNA at the 3′ or the 5′ end?	3′ end. Phosphate (PO_4) is at the 5′ end.
How many codons code for AAs? How many for *termination* of translation?	**61** codons code for **AAs** and **3** codons (**UAA, UGA, UAG**) code for the **termination** of translation.
What is the enzyme for the oxidative reaction in glycolysis?	Glyceraldehyde dehydrogenase
What substrate builds up in Tay-Sachs disease?	G_{M2} ganglioside
What pattern of genetic transmission is characterized by no transmission from M, maternal inheritance, and the potential for the disease to affect both sons and daughters of affected F?	Mitochondrial inheritance
What is the rate-limiting enzyme of glycogen synthesis?	Glycogen synthase
What sphingolipid is formed by the union of serine and palmitoyl CoA?	Sphingosine

What causes an increase in bone mineralization and Ca²⁺ along with PO₄ absorption from the GI tract and kidney tubules?

Vitamin D

What two sugars can be used to produce cerebrosides?

Glucose and galactose

What group of *eukaryotic* regulatory proteins has a major factor in controlling the gene expression embryonically?

Homeodomain proteins

What causes the lysis of RBCs by oxidizing agents in a G-6-PD deficiency?

The lack of glutathione peroxidase activity results in a decrease in NADPH production, leaving glutathione in the reduced state.

All AAs have titration plateaus at what pH values?

pH of 2 and 9

What cytoplasmic organelle carries the enzymes for elongation and desaturation of fatty acyl CoA?

SER

What is the binding site for RNA polymerase?

The **promoter** indicates where transcription will begin.

What vitamin is necessary for epithelial health?

Vitamin A is responsible for vision and epithelial health.

What lipoprotein is formed if an IDL particle acquires cholesterol from a HDL particle?

LDL

What structure of a protein describes the interaction among subunits?

Quaternary structure

What is the only factor of enzyme kinetics that the enzyme affects?

Ea (activation energy)

Is the Lac operon activated or inactivated in the presence of both glucose and lactose?

Inactivated; glucose results in decreased cAMP levels and therefore blocks protein binding between cAMP and CAP.

At the end of each round of β-oxidation, what is released?

Acetyl CoA, FADH, and NADH

What is the rate-limiting enzyme on glycolysis?

PFK-1 and **costs 1 ATP**

What enzyme of heme synthesis is deficient in the autosomal dominant disorder acute intermittent porphyria?

Uroporphyrinogen-I synthase

What enzyme is blocked by disulfiram?

Aldehyde dehydrogenase

Deficiencies in what enzyme result in insoluble glycogen synthesis formation?

α-1,6 transferase

What *eukaryotic translation* enzyme is associated with the following:

    Initiation

eIF-2 in the P site

    Elongation

eEF-1

    Termination

No enzymes are needed. When the stop codon reaches the A site, it results in termination.

What AA undergoes *N*-glycosylation?

Asparagine

What is the pyrimidine intermediate that joins PRPP?

Orotic acid

What intermediate of cholesterol synthesis anchors proteins in the membranes and forms CoA?

Farnesyl pyrophosphate (FPP)

What AA is a phenol?

Tyrosine

What hormone is activated in adipose tissue when blood glucose levels decrease?

Hormone-sensitive lipase

How many NADPHs are used per addition of acetyl CoA into a fatty acid chain?

2 NADPHs per acetyl CoA

What factors are needed for elongation in eukaryotes?

EF-1 and GTP

What purine base is contained in inosine monophosphate?

Hypoxanthine (remember, IMP is a precursor for AMP and GMP)

What are the two ways that nitrogen can enter into the urea cycle?

Aspartate and carbomoyl PO_4

What two requirements must be met for the Lac operon to be activated?

Lactose must be **present** and **glucose** must be **absent**

Name the phase of the eukaryotic cell cycle:

Period of cellular growth (translation and transcription) *before* DNA synthesis

G1 phase (gap 1)

Period of cellular growth (translation and transcription) *after* **DNA synthesis**	G2 phase (gap 2)
Period of DNA replication (preparing for mitosis)	S phase
Cells cease replicating (i.e., nerve cell)	G0 phase
True or false? RBCs *anaerobically* **use glucose in both the well-fed and fasting states.**	True. Remember, RBCs do **not** contain **mitochondria,** so they **cannot** metabolize **aerobically**.
What enzyme of the TCA cycle catalyzes the substrate level phosphorylation?	Succinyl CoA synthetase
What apoprotein on HDL activates lecithin–cholesterol acyltransferase (LCAT)?	apo A-1
What three AAs are used to synthesize the purine ring?	1. Glycine 2. Aspartate 3. Glutamine
How many ATPs are produced from cytoplasmic NADH oxidation using the *glycerol phosphate shuttle*?	2 ATPs by oxidative phosphorylation
What enzyme is deficient in patients with PKU?	Phenylalanine hydroxylase
What three steps of the TCA cycle generate NADH?	1. Malate dehydrogenase 2. Isocitrate dehydrogenase 3. α-Ketoglutarate dehydrogenase
What two enzymes of heme synthesis are inhibited by lead?	ALA dehydrogenase and ferrochelatase

What enzyme, induced by insulin and activated by apo C-II, is required for chylomicron and VLDL metabolism?

Lipoprotein lipase

What is the most common genetic deficiency resulting in hemolytic anemia?

G-6-PD deficiency; pyruvate kinase deficiency is second.

Are the following conditions associated with a negative or positive nitrogen balance?

   AA deficiency

Negative

   Growth

Positive

   Pregnancy

Positive

   Uncontrolled DM

Negative

   Starvation

Negative

   Infection

Negative

   Recovery from injury

Positive

   Kwashiorkor

Negative

Why is the liver unable to metabolize ketone bodies?

Hepatocytes lack the enzyme succinyl CoA acetoacetyl CoA transferase (thiophorase).

What toxin ADP-ribosylates via G_s protein to increase cAMP?

Cholera toxin

What two vitamins are inactivated when they come in contact with acetaldehyde?

Thiamine and folate

Name the end product or products:

Fatty acid synthesis	Palmitate
Fatty acid oxidation	Acetyl CoA and propionyl CoA (in odd chain fatty acids)

What is the term for production of a DNA copy from an RNA molecule?

Reverse transcription

What two monosaccharides are produced when lactose is hydrolyzed?

Galactose and glucose

What mineral is required for cross-linking of collagen molecules into fibrils?

The enzyme lysyl oxidase requires Cu^{2+} and O_2 to function properly.

What blotting technique uses the following for analysis?

DNA	Southern blot
Protein	Western blot
RNA	Northern blot

How many high-energy bonds does the cycle of elongation cost?

Four high energy bonds, two from ATP in AA activation and two from GTP

What enzyme of purine synthesis is inhibited by allopurinol and 6-mercaptopurine?

PRPP aminotransferase

True or false? The urea cycle takes place in both the cytoplasm and the mitochondria.

True. Remember, carbamoyl phosphate synthetase and ornithine transcarbamoylase are mitochondrial enzymes.

What is the only fatty acid that is gluconeogenic?	Propionic acid
What enzyme has a 5′ to 3′ synthesis of the Okazaki fragments, 3′ exonuclease activity, and 5′ exonuclease activity?	DNA polymerase I
In what organelle does the TCA cycle occur?	Mitochondria
Do genomic or cDNA libraries contain introns, exons, promoters, enhancers, and are they fragmented?	Genomic libraries are made from nuclear DNA, are fragmented, and contain all sequences found in the particular genome copied.
What enzyme is deficient in selective T cell immunodeficiency?	Purine nucleoside phosphorylase
True or false? Adipose tissue lacks glycerol kinase.	True. Adipose depends on glucose uptake for dihydroxyacetone phosphate (DHAP) production for triglyceride synthesis.
In what form is excess folate stored in the body?	N-5-methyl THF
What is the term for taking an mRNA molecule and arranging the AA sequence forming a protein?	Translation
What enzyme is blocked by hydroxyurea?	Ribonucleotide reductase
What protein carries free fatty acids to the liver?	Albumin
What substrate is built up in Niemann-Pick disease?	Sphingomyelin

True or false? Methylation of bacterial DNA *prevents* restriction endonuclease from cutting its own chromosomes.

True. Restriction endonucleases cut only *unmethylated* DNA.

What two AAs have a pKa of 10?

Lysine and tyrosine

What is the only enzyme in the body that uses N-5-methyl folate?

Homocysteine methyl transferase

How can you differentiate vitamin K from vitamin C deficiency by bleeding time and PT levels?

Vitamin **K** deficiency has **normal bleeding time** and **increased PT**, and vitamin **C** deficiency has **increased bleeding time** and **normal PT.**

What is the term for a unit of DNA that encodes a particular protein or RNA molecule?

A gene (a rather simple definition but accurate)

Is the coding or the template strand of DNA identical to mRNA (excluding the T/U difference)?

The **coding strand** is identical to mRNA, and the template strand is complementary and antiparallel.

What enzyme is deficient in acute intermittent porphyria?

Uroporphyrinogen I synthetase

What five cofactors and coenzymes are required by pyruvate dehydrogenase?

1. TTP
2. Lipoic acid
3. Coenzyme A from pantothenate
4. NAD(H) (from niacin or tryptophan)
5. $FADH_2$ (from riboflavin)

What pattern of genetic transmission affects only M and has no M-to-M transmission, and mother is usually an unaffected carrier?

X-linked recessive

To what does aldose reductase convert galactose?

Galactitol

Name three *purine* bases that are *not* found in nucleic acids.

Xanthine, hypoxanthine, theophylline, theobromine, caffeine, and uric acid are all purines.

What water-soluble-vitamin deficiency is associated with cheilosis and *magenta tongue*?

Riboflavin (B_2)

What is the precursor of all sphingolipids?

Ceramide

What three substances stimulate glycogenolysis?

1. Ca^{2+}: calmodulin ratio
2. Epinephrine
3. Glucagon

What is the primer for the synthesis of the second strand in production of cDNA from mRNA?

The **hairpin loop** made by reverse transcriptase at the $3'$ end of the first strand is the primer.

What factors are needed for elongation in prokaryotes?

EF-Tu or EF-ts and GTP

What restriction endonuclease site is destroyed in sickle β-globin allele?

*Mst*II; changing **codon 6** (from A to T) destroys the restriction site.

What complex is needed for propionyl CoA carboxylase?

Biotin, ATP, and CO_2

What enzyme catalyzes the reversible oxidative deamination of glutamate and produces the TCA cycle intermediate α-ketoglutarate?

Glutamate dehydrogenase

What enzyme is deficient in congenital erythropoietic porphyria?	Uroporphyrinogen III cosynthase
What is the drug of choice for treating a patient with hyperuricemia due to *overproduction* of uric acid?	Allopurinol
What is the maximum rate possible with a given amount of enzyme?	V_{max}
From what do catalase, superoxide dismutase, and glutathione peroxidase defend the cell?	Production of oxygen free radicals
What signals are used to direct an enzyme to a lysosome?	Phosphorylation of mannose residues
What enzyme catalyzes the rate-limiting step of the urea cycle?	Carbamoyl phosphate synthetase I
What liver enzyme, for triglyceride synthesis, converts glycerol to glycerol-3-phosphate?	Glycerol kinase
What *organ* functions to keep blood glucose levels normal through both well-fed and fasting states and produces ketones in response to increased fatty acid oxidation?	Liver
What pattern of inheritance does G-6-PD deficiency follow?	X-linked recessive

What is the term for conversion of a dsDNA molecule to the base sequence of an ssRNA molecule?	Transcription (**C** comes before **L** in the alphabet, and transCription comes before transLation)
Via what cell surface receptor does HDL cholesterol from the periphery enter hepatoceles?	Scavenger receptor (SR-B1)
Which shuttle is used to bring fatty acyl CoA from the cytoplasm for ketogenesis?	Carnitine acyl CoA transferase II
What enzyme is blocked by 5-FU?	Thymidylate synthetase
What disease has a genetically low level of UDPglucuronate transferase, resulting in elevated free unconjugated bilirubin?	Gilbert's syndrome
What AA has a pKa of 13?	Arginine
What X-*linked recessive* disorder is characterized by hyperuricemia, spastic cerebral palsy, mental retardation, and self-mutilation?	Lesch-Nyhan syndrome
How many ATPs per glucose are generated from glycolysis in RBCs?	**2 ATPs,** because RBCs use only anaerobic metabolism.
What enzyme catalyzes the rate-limiting step in glycogenolysis?	Glycogen phosphorylase

Would a G-C or an A-T rich dsDNA sequence have a higher melting point? Why?	**G-C rich** sequences, because they have **3 hydrogen bonds,** where **A-T** has **2 hydrogen bonds,** resulting in higher melting points.
As what AAs do muscles send nitrogen to the liver?	Alanine and glutamine
What sphingolipid cannot be produced without sialic acid and amino sugars?	Ganglioside
What happens to affinity if you increase K_m?	Affinity decreases; they are inversely proportional.
What type of bilirubin is found in neonatal jaundice?	Indirect or unconjugated
What two AAs do not have more than one codon?	Methionine (start) and tryptophan are the only two AAs with only one codon.
What bonds are broken by *exonucleases*?	**External** 3′,5′ PDE bonds
How can a genetic deficiency of carbamoyl phosphate synthetase be differentiated from an ornithine transcarbamoylase deficiency?	Uracil and orotic acid levels **increase** with **ornithine transcarbamoylase deficiency** and are normal in carbamoyl phosphate synthetase deficiency.
Name the lipoprotein based on the following characteristics.	
apo E	IDL
apo B-100	LDL
apo E, apo B-100, apo C-II	VLDL

apo A-1, apo E, apo C-II	HDL
apo E, apo C-II, apoB-48	Chylomicrons
True or false? There is no hormonal control to the TCA cycle.	True. The energy status of the cell dictates if the cycle is running or relaxing.
What are the three tissues where triacylglycerols are produced?	1. Liver 2. Muscle 3. Adipose tissue
What toxin ADP-ribosylates via G_i to increase cAMP?	Pertussis toxin
What enzyme catalyzes the rate-limiting step in heme synthesis?	δ-ALA synthase
What cycle is responsible for converting to glucose in the liver the lactate produced in the RBCs?	Cori cycle
What enzyme is used to remove the hairpin loop during production of cDNA from mRNA?	S1 nuclease
Does a saturated fatty acid have double bonds?	No, unsaturated fatty acids have double bonds.

What *pyrimidine* base is found

Only in RNA?	Uracil
Only in DNA?	Thymine
In both DNA and RNA?	Cytosine
What two AAs require vitamin C for hydroxylation?	Proline and lysine

What is the only organ in the body that can produce ketone bodies?

The liver (in the mitochondria)

What determines the rate of reaction?

The energy of activation

What is the term for the number of trinucleotide repeats increasing with successive generations and correlating with increased severity of disease?

Anticipation, associated with fragile X syndrome; Huntington's disease is also associated with a decrease in onset of age.

What enzyme is blocked by methotrexate/ trimethoprim?

Dihydrofolate reductase

What fructose metabolism enzyme is deficient in patients with vomiting, apathy, diarrhea, jaundice, proximal renal tubular acidosis, hypoglycemia, and hyperuricemia?

Aldolase B deficiencies are treated by eliminating fructose from the diet.

What enzyme catalyzes the rate-limiting step in purine synthesis?

PRPP aminotransferase

What water-soluble-vitamin deficiency is associated with poor wound healing, easy bruising, bleeding gums, anemia, and painful glossitis?

Vitamin C

What three substrates control the enzyme PEPCK for the conversion of OAA to pyruvate in the cytoplasm?

1. Cortisol (stimulates PEPCK)
2. Glucagon
3. GTP

What genetic defect is characterized by coarse facial features, gingival hyperplasia, macroglossia, psychomotor and growth retardation, club foot, claw hand, cardiorespiratory failure, and death in the first decade of life?

I-cell disease is a result of a genetic defect affecting the phosphorylation of mannose residues.

What two glycolytic enzymes catalyze the *substrate-level phosphorylations?*

3-Phosphoglycerate kinase and pyruvate kinase; this **produces two ATPs per enzyme (total four ATPs)**

What pathway uses HMG CoA synthetase in the cytoplasm?

Cholesterol biosynthesis

Where in the body is heme converted to bilirubin?

RES

What protein is required by *prokaryotic* RNA polymerases to initiate transcription at the promoter region of DNA?

Sigma factor

What enzyme catalyzes the rate-limiting step in pyrimidine synthesis?

Aspartate transcarbamylase

What are the two actions of calcitonin?

It increases Ca^{2+} excretion from the kidney and increases bone mineralization.

What enzyme of the purine salvage pathway is deficient in the following?

Selective T-cell immunodeficiency

Purine nucleoside phosphorylase

SCID

Adenosine deaminase

Lesch-Nyhan syndrome	HGPRT
In what cycle does glucose go to the muscle, where it is converted to pyruvate and then into alanine before being taken back to the liver?	Alanine cycle
What is the primary end product of pyrimidine synthesis?	UMP
What *pyrimidine* base is produced by deaminating cytosine?	Uracil
What AA is classified as *basic* even though its pK is 6.5 to 7?	Histidine, because of the imidazole ring found in the R group, is basic.
What enzyme is deficient in hereditary protoporphyria?	Ferrochelatase
What elongation factor is inactivated by ADP ribosylation, preventing translation?	eEF-2 is the site where *Pseudomonas* and *Diphtheria* toxins work.
Is linolenic acid an omega-3 or omega-6 fatty acid?	Omega-3; linoleic is omega-6
How many ATPs per glucose are generated in *glycolysis*?	**8 ATPs if aerobic, 2 ATPs if anaerobic** (6 ATPs + 2 ATPs + 2 ATPs − 2 ATPs = 8 ATPs)
Name the three ketone bodies.	Acetoacetate, acetone, and β-hydroxybutyrate
What three bases are pyrimidines?	1. Cytosine 2. Uracil (only in RNA) 3. Thymidine

Name the RNA subtype based on the following:

The most abundant form of RNA in the cell	rRNA
Found only in the nucleus of *eukaryotes* and functions to remove introns from mRNA	snRNA
Only type of RNA that is translated	mRNA
Carries AA to the ribosome for protein synthesis	tRNA
RNA molecules with enzymatic activity	Ribozymes
Found only in the nucleus of eukaryotic cells and are precursors of mRNA	hnRNA

What enzyme is deficient in the following glycogen storage diseases?

von Gierke's disease	Glucose-6-phosphatase
Pompe's disease	**Lysosomal** α-1,4-glucosidase
McArdle's disease	**Muscle** glycogen phosphorylase
Hers' disease	**Hepatic** glycogen phosphorylase

In *prokaryotes*, what is the term for a set of structural genes that code for a select group of proteins and the regulatory elements required for the expression of such gene?	Operon

What are the two most common AAs found in histones?

Lysine and arginine

What five pathways use SAM (S-adenosylmethionine) as the methyl donor?

1. Epinephrine synthesis
2. Phosphatidyl choline
3. Creatine
4. Methylation of cytosine
5. N-methyl cap of mRNA

What complex of the ETC contains Cu $^{2+}$?

Complex 4

How many ATPs per glucose are produced by pyruvate dehydrogenase?

6 ATPs (remember **2 pyruvates** per glucose are produced, and **2 NADHs** result from production of acetyl CoA, so 6 ATPs)

What is the size of the prokaryotic ribosome?

70S ribosomes in **prokaryotes** and 80S ribosomes in eukaryotes

What type of fatty acid is associated with a decrease in serum triglycerides and cardiovascular disease?

Omega-3 fatty acids

What disease is produced by a deficiency in the enzyme tyrosinase?

Albinism. Tyrosine is converted to melanin by the enzyme tyrosinase.

In what form are triglycerides sent to adipose tissue from the liver?

VLDLs

What determines the rate of a reaction?

The energy of activation (Ea)

What is the rate-limiting enzyme of the HMP shunt?

G-6-PD

What vitamin is necessary for the transfer of one amino group from a carbon skeleton to another?

Pyridoxal phosphate is derived from **vitamin B$_6$** and is needed to transfer the amino groups of one carbon skeleton to another.

What is the only sphingolipid that contains choline and PO$_4$?	Sphingomyelin (lecithin also, but it is not a sphingolipid)
What protein catalyzes the formation of the last PDE bond between the Okazaki fragments to produce a continuous strand?	DNA ligase
What type of damage to the kidneys is caused by drinking ethylene glycol (antifreeze)?	Nephrotoxic oxylate stones
What water-soluble-vitamin deficiency may result from eating *raw eggs*?	Biotin (only if eaten in large quantities)
Regarding the Lac operon, for what do the following genes code?	
Z gene	β-Galactosidase
Y gene	Galactoside permease
I gene	Lac repressor protein
A gene	Thiogalactoside transacetylase
What attaches to protons and allows them to enter into the mitochondria without going through the ATP-generating system?	2,4-Dinitrophenol
1-α-Hydroxylase activity is increased in response to what two physiologic states? (hint: think of vitamin D activity)	**Hypo**calcemia and **hypo**phosphatemia

What is the major ketone body produced during alcoholic ketoacidosis?	β-Hydroxybutyrate
What enzyme catalyzes the rate-limiting step in the TCA cycle?	Isocitrate dehydrogenase
Name the pattern of genetic transmission characterized thus: both M and F are affected; M may transmit to M; each generation has at least one affected parent; and one mutant allele may produce the disease.	Autosomal dominant
What bonds are broken by *endonucleases*?	**Internal** 3′, 5′ PDE bonds
Name the GLUT transporter based on the following:	
Found in liver and pancreatic β-cells	GLUT 2
Found in skeletal muscle and adipose tissues	GLUT 4
Found in most tissues, including brain and RBCs	GLUT 3 and 4
What enzyme catalyzes the rate-limiting step in fatty acid oxidation?	Carnitine acyltransferase-I
What enzyme of the TCA cycle also acts as complex II of the ETC?	Succinate dehydrogenase

What is the term for chemicals that keep the pH constant despite the formation of acids and bases during metabolism?

Buffers (remember that buffers are best when they are used in a pH range near its pK)

In the mitochondria, what complex is needed for pyruvate carboxylase to catalyze the reaction from pyruvate to OAA?

Biotin, ATP, and CO_2

How many ATPs are produced from cytoplasmic NADH oxidation using the *malate shuttle*?

3 ATPs by oxidative phosphorylation

What is the rate-limiting step of the following?

Fatty acid synthesis

Acetyl CoA carboxylase

β-Oxidation

Carnitine acyltransferase I

Ketogenolysis

HMG CoA synthase

Cholesterol synthesis

HMG CoA reductase

What direction does RNA polymerase move along the template strand of DNA during transcription?

3′-5′ direction, synthesizing RNA in the 5′-3′ direction

True or false? Histidine activates the histidine operon.

False. Histidine operon is **activated** when there are **low** intracellular levels of **histidine**.

What *organ* is responsible for the elimination of excess nitrogen from the body?

The **kidneys** excrete the excess nitrogen from the body as urea in the urine.

What is the only way to increase maximum velocity (V_{max})?

Increase enzyme concentrations

Name the two *purine* bases found in both DNA and RNA.

Adenine and guanine

What *prokaryotic* positioning enzyme in *translation* is blocked by the following?

    Tetracycline

eEF-Tu and eEF-Ts of the 30S ribosomal subunit

    Erythromycin

eEF-G of the 50S subunit

    Streptomycin

eIF-2 of the 30S subunit

True or false? DNA polymerases can correct mistakes, whereas RNA polymerases lack this ability.

True. DNA polymerases have 3'-5' exonuclease activity for proofreading.

What are the two precursors of heme?

Glycine and succinyl-CoA

What two factors cause PTH to be secreted?

A decrease in Ca^{2+} and a decrease in PO_4

What are the nonoxidative enzymes of the HMP shunt? Are the reactions they catalyze reversible or irreversible?

Transketolase and transaldolase. The reactions they catalyze are reversible.

What are the five AAs that are both *ketogenic and glucogenic*?

Isoleucine, threonine, tryptophan, tyrosine, and phenylalanine

What artificial sweetener must patients with PKU avoid?

Aspartame

Cri-du-chat syndrome results in a terminal deletion of the short arm of what chromosome?

Chromosome 5

What substrate gets built up in Gaucher's disease?

Glucosyl cerebroside

What protein prevents ssDNA from reannealing during DNA replication?

Single-strand DNA binding protein

What type of jaundice is seen in Dubin-Johnson syndrome?

Conjugated (direct) hyperbilirubinemia, a transport defect

What type of DNA library is made from the mRNA from a tissue expressing a particular gene?

cDNA libraries are derived from mRNA, are continuous, and contain no introns or regulatory elements.

What is the most common cause of vitamin B_6 deficiency?

Isoniazid treatment

What lysosomal enzyme is deficient in

    Gaucher's disease?

Glucocerebrosidase

    Niemann-Pick disease?

Sphingomyelinase

    Tay-Sachs disease?

Hexosaminidase A

What are the three exceptions to the rule of codominant gene expression?

Barr bodies in females, T-cell receptor loci, and immunoglobulin light and heavy chain loci

How many kilocalories per gram are produced from the degradation of fat? CHO? Protein?

9 kcal/g from **fat** metabolism; **4** kcal/g from both **CHO** and **protein** metabolism

What is the only way to increase the V_{max} of a reaction?

Increase the concentration of enzymes

From which two substances are phospholipids made?

Diacylglycerols and phosphatidic acid

What intermediate enables propionyl CoA to enter into the TCA cycle?

Succinyl CoA

What vitamin is an important component of rhodopsin?

Vitamin A

What is the term to describe the 5′-3′ sequence of one strand being the same as the opposite 5′-3′ strand?

Palindrome

What gluconeogenic enzyme is absent in muscle, accounting for its inability to use glycogen as a source for blood glucose?

Glucose-6-phosphatase

What is the term for vitamin D deficiency *prior to* epiphyseal fusion?

Rickets prior to fusion, osteomalacia if the deficiency occurs **after** epiphyseal fusion.

In what disease is there a genetic absence of UDPglucuronate transferase, resulting in an increase in free unconjugated bilirubin?

Crigler-Najjar syndrome

What enzyme requires molybdenum as a cofactor?	Xanthine oxidase
At what three sites can the HMP shunt enter into glycolysis?	1. Fructose-6-phosphate 2. Glucose-6-phosphate 3. Glyceraldehyde-3-phosphate
What is the term for the pH range where the dissociation of H$^+$occurs?	pK (think of it as where half is base and half is acid)
What regulates the rate of ketone body formation?	The rate of β-oxidation
What are the eight liver-specific enzymes?	1. Fructokinase 2. Glucokinase 3. Glycerol kinase 4. PEPCK 5. Pyruvate carboxylase 6. Galactokinase 7. Fructose-1,6-biphosphate 8. Glucose-6-phosphate
How many bases upstream is the *eukaryotic* TATA box promoter?	There are two eukaryotic upstream promoters. The TATA box is **−25 base pairs upstream;** the CAAT box is −75 bases upstream.
What is needed to initiate translation?	IF and GTP (eIF for eukaryotes)
What part of the 30S ribosome binds to the Shine-Dalgarno sequence?	16S subunit
What component of the ETC is inhibited by the following?	
Barbiturates	Complex I
Antimycin A	Cytochrome b/c1

Cyanide	Cytochrome a/a3
Oligomycin	Fo/F1 complex
Atractyloside	ATP/ADP Translocase
CO	Cytochrome a/a3
Rotenone	Complex I
Azide	Cytochrome a/a3

What AA is a precursor of the following substances?

Serotonin	Tryptophan
GABA	Glutamate
Histamine	Histidine
Creatine	Glycine/arginine
NAD	Tryptophan
N_2O	Arginine

What two enzymes are vitamin B_{12}–dependent?

Homocysteine methyl transferase and methylmalonyl CoA transferase

What two post-transcriptional enzymes in collagen synthesis require ascorbic acid to function properly?

Prolyl and lysyl hydroxylases

What three organs participate in production of vitamin D?

1. Skin
2. Liver
3. Kidney

What water-soluble-vitamin deficiency is associated with *neural tube defects* in the fetus?

Folic acid

What phase of Interphase is *haploid* (N)?

G1 phase; G2 and S phase are **diploid** (2N).

What neurotransmitter inhibits the optic nerve bipolar cell and shuts off in response to light?

Glutamate

Which of the following—DNA methylating enzymes, scaffolding proteins, histone acetylases, or deacetylases—is a regulator of eukaryotic gene expression?

Histone acetylases is a *regulator* favoring gene expression. All of the **others** favor *inactivation*.

Name the pattern of genetic transmission characterized thus: both M and F affected; no M-to-M transmission; affected M passes trait to all daughters, every generation; affected F passes trait to both sons and daughters; a single mutant allele can produce the disease.

X-linked dominant

What fat-soluble vitamin is connected to selenium metabolism?

Vitamin E

Why are eukaryotes unable to perform transcription and translation at the same time like prokaryotes?

In eukaryotes **transcription** occurs in the **nucleus** and **translation** in the **cytoplasm**.

What is determined by the secondary structure of an AA?

The folding of an AA chain

What three vitamin deficiencies are associated with homocystinemia?

Folate, vitamin B_{12}, and vitamin B_6

If the pH is *more acidic* than the pI, does the protein carry a net positive or net negative charge?

When the pH is **more acidic** than the pI, it has a **net positive charge,** and when the pH is **more basic** than the pI, it has a **net negative charge.**

What form of continuous DNA, used in cloning, has no introns or regulatory elements?

cDNA, when it is made from mRNA

What is the *start codon,* and what does it code for in eukaryotes? Prokaryotes?

The one start codon, **AUG,** in *eukaryotes* codes for **methionine** and in *prokaryotes* **formylmethionine.**

What parasite found in *raw fish* can produce vitamin B_{12} deficiency?

Diphyllobothrium latum

Methylating uracil produces what *pyrimidine* base?

Thymine

Name the *eukaryotic* RNA polymerase based on the following:

Synthesizes tRNA, snRNA, and the 5S rRNA

RNA polymerase III

Synthesizes hnRNA, mRNA, and snRNA

RNA polymerase II

Synthesizes 28S, 18S and 5.8S rRNAs

RNA polymerase I

What is the primary *screening* test used to detect HIV-infected individuals? *Confirmatory* test?

ELISA is used as a *screening* test because it is very sensitive; **Western blot** is used as a *confirmatory* test because it detects antibodies (protein) to the HIV virus.

How many covalent bonds per purine-pyrimidine base pairing are broken during denaturation of dsDNA?

None. Denaturation of dsDNA breaks **hydrogen** bonds, not covalent bonds.

How many hydrogen bonds link A-T? C-G?

A-T are linked by 2 hydrogen bonds, C-G by 3 hydrogen bonds.

What DNA replication enzyme breaks the hydrogen bond of base pairing, forming two replication forks?

Helicase (requires ATP for energy)

4

Microbiology and Immunology

MICROBIOLOGY

What does *Candida albicans* do that distinguishes it from other fungi?

It forms a germinal tube at 37°C.

What protozoal parasite results in dysentery with blood and pus in the stool, is transmitted via fecal-oral route, is diagnosed by cysts or trophozoites in the stool, and forms liver abscesses and inverted flask-shaped lesions in the large intestine?

Entamoeba histolytica (treat with metronidazole)

What is the most likely causative organism for a patient with folliculitis after spending time in a *hot tub*?

Pseudomonas aeruginosa

What two viruses get their envelope not from budding but from coding?

HIV and poxvirus

Which type of hepatitis can cause hepatocellular carcinoma?

Hepatitis B

Gas gangrene is associated with which *Clostridium* species?

Clostridium perfringens

Which dimorphic fungus is found as hyphae with nondescript conidia in rotting wood in the Upper Great Lakes, Ohio, Mississippi, eastern seaboard of the United States, and southern Canada?

Blastomyces dermatitidis

Which parasitic organism, when it crosses the placenta, results in intracerebral calcifications, chorioretinitis, microcephaly, hydrocephaly, and convulsions?

Toxoplasma gondii

What staphylococcal species is positive for β-hemolysis and coagulase?

Staphylococcus aureus

What vector is associated with malaria?

Anopheles mosquito

What is the term for hyphae with constrictions at each septum that are commonly seen in *Candida albicans*?

Pseudohyphae

Which cestode infection results in *alveolar hydatid cyst disease*?

Echinococcus multilocularis

Which hepatitis virus is in the Flaviviridae family?

Hepatitis C

What nonmotile gram-negative, non–lactose-fermenting facultative anaerobic rod uses the human colon as its only reservoir and is transmitted by fecal-oral spread?

Shigella

What is the only *Rickettsia* that is stable in the environment?

Coxiella burnetii

Regarding the viral growth curve, is the internal virus present before or after the eclipse period?

After the **eclipse** period

What Ab is an indication of recurrent disease for hepatitis?

HB_c Ab

What small gram-positive, non–spore-forming rod is a facultative intracellular parasite that grows in the cold and is associated with unpasteurized milk products?

Listeria monocytogenes

What is the only DNA virus that is not icosahedral?

Poxvirus

Which organism causes trench mouth?

Fusobacterium

True or false? All of the following are inactivated vaccines available in the United States: influenza, *Vibrio cholera*, hepatitis A, rabies, and adenovirus.

False. Adenovirus vaccine is a live pathogenic virus in an enteric coated capsule. All of the others are inactivated vaccines.

Name the *Plasmodium* species based on the following information:

No persistent liver stage or relapse; blood smear shows multiple ring forms and crescent-shaped gametes; irregular febrile pattern; associated with cerebral malaria

Plasmodium falciparum

No persistent liver stage or relapse; blood smear shows rosette schizonts; 72-hour fever spike pattern	*Plasmodium malariae*
Persistent hypnozoite liver stage with relapses; blood smear shows amoeboid trophozoites with oval, jagged infected RBCs; 48-hour fever spike pattern	*Plasmodium ovale*
Persistent hypnozoite liver stage with relapses; blood smear shows amoeboid trophozoites; 48-hour fever spike pattern; the most prevalent form worldwide	*Plasmodium vivax*
True or false? A positive PPD skin test indicates the patient has active pulmonary disease.	False. The PPD tests exposure to TB.
What *viral* infection is known to cause intracerebral calcifications?	CMV; *Toxoplasma* also causes intracerebral calcifications but it is a parasite.
What viruses are associated with cervical carcinoma?	HPVs 16 and 18
What motile, gram-negative spiral bacillus with flagella is oxidase positive, urease positive, and associated with gastritis, peptic ulcer disease, and stomach cancer?	*Helicobacter pylori*
What glycoprotein in the HIV virus is used for fusion?	GP41

What Ag is needed to diagnose an infectious patient with hepatitis B?	HB_eAg
Which organism causes multiple infections by antigen switching?	*Borrelia recurrentis*
What is the first Ag seen in an individual with hepatitis?	HB_sAg (incubation period)
With which DNA virus are Guarnieri bodies associated?	Variola (smallpox)
What nematode is known as *pinworms*? What is the treatment?	*Enterobius vermicularis;* the treatment is albendazole.
What protein allows *Mycoplasma* to attach to the respiratory epithelium?	P1 protein
What organism is associated with the following types of diarrhea?	
Day care–associated diarrhea in infants	Rotavirus
Watery diarrhea from beef, poultry, or gravies	*Clostridium perfringens*
Rice water stools	*Vibrio cholera*
Diarrhea associated with raw or undercooked shellfish	*Vibrio parahaemolyticus*
Bloody diarrhea associated with hamburger ingestion	Enterotoxigenic *Escherichia coli*

Which fungus is found worldwide on plants, is a cigar-shaped yeast in tissue form, and results in rose gardener's disease?	*Sporothrix schenckii*
Which type of hepatitis is a picornavirus?	Hepatitis A (infectious)
What gram-positive rod is distinguished by its tumbling motility?	*Listeria*
What is the vector for *Leishmania* infections?	The sandfly
What is the term of the viral growth period when no viruses can be found intracellularly?	Eclipse period
What organism causes Q fever?	*Coxiella burnetii*
What are the three naked RNA viruses?	1. **P**icornavirus 2. **C**alicivirus 3. **R**eovirus (Remember **PCR**)
HIV's capsid, core nucleocapsid, and matrix proteins are products of what structural gene?	*gag* gene
What facultative intracellular fungus is associated with hepatosplenomegaly?	*Histoplasma capsulatum* infects the cells of the RES and can result in hepatosplenomegaly.
What type of hepatitis has the highest mortality rate among pregnant women?	Hepatitis E

Which gram-negative diplococcus ferments maltose?

Meningococcus (*Gonococcus* does not)

Are antibiotics helpful in treating a disease caused by a prion?

No. Prions are infectious proteins, so antibiotics are useless.

What bacterium is responsible for woolsorter's disease?

Bacillus anthracis

What picornavirus is associated with hand-foot-and-mouth disease?

Coxsackie A

What is the only trematode that is not hermaphroditic?

Schistosoma have separate males and females.

What water-associated organism is a weakly stained gram-negative rod that requires cysteine and iron for growth?

Legionella (think air conditioners)

With what virus are Downey type II cells associated?

EBV

True or false? Interferons are eukaryotic proteins that inhibit viral replication by being virus specific.

False. Interferons are produced by virally infected cells to **inhibit** viral replication via RNA endonucleases. They **do not** act directly on the virus, nor are they virus specific.

What is the vector for yellow fever?

Aedes mosquito

What small, facultative gram-negative intracellular rod's transmission is associated with unpasteurized dairy products and undulant fever?

Brucella

True or false? All *Proteus* species are urease positive.

True

Which genus of dermatophytes is associated with the following sites of infection?

    Nails and skin only

Epidermophyton

    Hair and skin only

Microsporum

    Skin, hair, and nails

Trichophyton

What protein of the HIV virus does ELISA detect to determine whether a patient is HIV positive?

P24

What genus of bacteria is described by catalase-positive, gram-positive cocci in clusters?

Staphylococcus

True or false? *Vibrio parahaemolyticus* require NaCl in its growth medium.

True. *Staphylococcus aureus* and group D enterococci also grow in high-salt media.

What virus causes small pink benign wartlike tumors and is associated with HIV-positive patients?

Molluscum contagiosum

What two bacteria are associated with drinking unpasteurized milk?

Brucella and *Listeria* (has tumbling motility)

What cestode causes *cysticercosis*?

Taenia solium

What DNA virus is associated with exanthem subitum (roseola)?

HHV 6

Which acid-fast rod is an obligate intracellular parasite?

Mycobacterium leprae

What form of the *Plasmodium* species is ingested by mosquitoes?

Gametocytes

What small gram-negative aerobic rod requires Regan-Lowe or Bordet-Gengou medium for growth?

Bordetella pertussis

True or false? *Streptococci* have catalase.

False. Staphylococci have catalase; *streptococci* do not.

What three bacteria are positive to quellung reactive test?

1. *Neisseria meningitidis*
2. *Haemophilus influenzae*
3. *Streptococcus pneumoniae*

A patient goes to the ER with abdominal cramps, vomiting, diarrhea, and sweating less than 24 hours after eating potato salad at a picnic; what is the most likely responsible organism?

Staphylococcus aureus

True or false? All spore formers are gram positive.

True

What is the only DNA virus that has the reverse transcriptase enzyme?

Hepadnavirus

What enzyme does HIV use to integrate the proviral dsDNA into the host?

Integrase

What are the two hepatitis viruses that can be chronic and can lead eventually to hepatocellular carcinoma?

Hepatitis B and hepatitis C

What gram-positive spore-forming anaerobic rod blocks the release of ACh at the NMJ, resulting in reversible flaccid paralysis?

Clostridium botulinum

Name at least two products of HIV's *pol* gene.

Protease, integrase, and reverse transcriptase

What form of *Plasmodium* species affects the liver?

Hypnozoite

What small coagulase-positive, gram-negative rod with bipolar staining is a facultative intracellular parasite resulting in buboes?

Yersinia pestis

What hemoflagellate species is the cause of Chagas disease?

Trypanosoma cruzi

To what host cell receptor does the rabies virus attach?

ACh receptor

Which hepatitis virus is in the Picornaviridae family?

Hepatitis A

Abs to what hepatitis B Ag provide immunity?

Abs to HB_sAg

What type of spore is defined as an asexual budding daughter yeast cell?

Blastoconidia

Which of the following characteristics accurately describe fungi, bacteria, viruses, and parasites?

Eukaryotic cell, 15 to 25 microns, 80S ribosomes, no cell walls, replicates via cytokinesis with mitosis and meiosis	Parasites
Small prokaryotic cells; no histones; 70S ribosomes; no sterols in cell membrane; peptidoglycans in cell wall; replicate by binary fission	Bacteria
Eukaryotic cell; 3 to 10 microns; 80S ribosomes; chitinous cell wall; ergosterol in cell membrane; replicate via cytokinesis with mitosis and meiosis	Fungi
Acellular; some are enveloped; replicate within the host cell; no cell walls	Viruses

What mosquito is the vector for dengue fever?   *Aedes* (the same for yellow fever)

True or false? *Gonococcus* **is encapsulated.**   False. *Meningococcus* is encapsulated; *Gonococcus* is not.

What virus is associated with Guarnieri bodies?   Variola virus

Regarding the viral growth curve, is the external virus present before or after the latent period?   **After** the **latent** period

What aerobic branching rod that is gram positive and partially acid-fast is associated with cavitary bronchopulmonary disease in immunosuppressed patients?

Nocardia asteroides

What obligate extracellular fungus is silver stain–positive and is associated with pneumonia in patients with AIDS?

Pneumocystis carinii

What Vi-encapsulated gram-negative motile anaerobic rod that produces H2S is associated with enteric fever, gastroenteritis, and septicemia?

Salmonella typhi

What is the most likely organism causing cellulitis in a patient who was cut by an *oyster shell*?

Vibrio vulnificus

What virus is associated with the Norwalk agent?

Calicivirus

Describe the organism based on the following information:

    β-Hemolytic *Streptococcus*; positive cAMP test; hydrolyzes hippurate

Streptococcus agalactiae

    β-Hemolytic *Streptococcus*; lysed by bile; sensitive to Optochin

Pneumococcus (*Streptococcus pneumoniae*)

β-hemolytic
Streptococcus; not lysed
by bile; not sensitive to
Optochin

Streptococcus viridans

β-hemolytic
Streptococcus sensitive
to bacitracin

Streptococcus pyogenes

**What is the only nonmotile
pathogenic *Clostridium*
species?**

Clostridium perfringens

**If a virus has positive sense
RNA, can it be used as
mRNA or is a template
needed?**

Positive sense RNA **can be used as
mRNA**. Negative sense RNA **cannot** be
used as mRNA; it requires special
RNA-dependent RNA polymerases.

**Where do adult tapeworms
develop, in the intermediate
or definitive host?**

Adult tapeworms develop in the
definitive host, whereas **cysticerci** or
larvae develop in the **intermediate host**.

**Which streptococcal species
is characterized by being
catalase negative, turning
bile esculin agar black,
producing a positive PYR
test, and resulting in biliary
and urinary tract
infections?**

Enterococcus (*Streptococcus faecalis*)

**What three carcinomas are
associated with EBV?**

1. Burkitt's lymphoma
2. Nasopharyngeal carcinoma
3. Thymic carcinoma

**Which organism causes
trench fever?**

Rochalimaea quintana

**Based on the onset of the
symptoms, how are
bacterial conjunctivitis
from *Neisseria* and
Chlamydia differentiated?**

The onset of symptoms for *Neisseria
gonorrhea* conjunctivitis is **2 to 5 days,**
whereas onset of symptoms for
Chlamydia trachomatis is **5 to 10 days**.

What toxin, produced by *Clostridium tetani*, binds to ganglioside receptors and blocks the release of glycine and GABA at the spinal synapse?

Tetanospasmin (also called tetanus toxin)

True or false? All of the following are *live attenuated vaccines* available in the United States: measles, mumps, varicella zoster, and *Francisella tularensis*.

True. So are rubeola, smallpox, yellow fever, and the Sabin polio vaccine.

What family do the following viruses belong to?

Ebola	Filovirus
California encephalitis	Bunyavirus
Hantavirus	Bunyavirus
Rabies	Rhabdovirus
RSV	Paramyxovirus
Measles	Paramyxovirus

What microaerophile is a motile gram-negative curved rod with polar flagella that causes infectious diarrhea at low doses (<500)?

Campylobacter jejuni

What bacterium is diagnosed using the *Dieterle* silver stain?

Legionella

How many strains of *Pneumococcus* capsular polysaccharides are present in the vaccine?

The vaccine contains 23 capsular polysaccharides.

What nematode is known as *whipworms*? What is the treatment?

Trichuris trichiura is treated with albendazole.

Which *Streptococcus pyogenes* toxin is immunogenic?

Streptolysin O

A urethral swab of a patient shows gram-negative diplococci in PMNs; what organism do you diagnose?

Neisseria gonorrhoeae

A suspected dermatophyte infection is stained with KOH. What spore type do you expect to see?

Arthroconidia with hyphae

What negative sense RNA virus is associated with cough, coryza, and conjunctivitis with photophobia?

Measles (rubeola)

Which M-protein strain of *Streptococcus pyogenes* is associated with acute glomerulonephritis?

M12 strains

What are the three C's of measles?

1. Cough
2. Coryza
3. Conjunctivitis

What is the term given to *arthropod-borne* viruses?

Arboviruses (bunyavirus, flavivirus, and togavirus)

Which organism causes Weil's disease?

Leptospira

What form of the *Plasmodium* species are injected into humans by mosquitoes?

Sporozoites

What ssDNA virus must make dsDNA before it makes mRNA?

Parvovirus (it is the only ssDNA virus)

What is the vector of African sleeping sickness?

The tsetse fly

What HIV enzyme produces a dsDNA provirus?

Reverse transcriptase

What non–spore-forming gram-positive aerobic rod produces bull neck, sore throat with pseudomembranes, myocarditis, and sometimes respiratory obstructions?

Corynebacterium diphtheriae

What organism is associated with megaloblastic anemia?

Diphyllobothrium latum

What is the most serious form of tinea capitis, which results in permanent hair loss and is highly contagious?

Tinea favosa (favus)

What are the first intermediate hosts for trematodes?

Snails

What are the four capsular polysaccharides used in the *Neisseria meningitides* vaccine?

Y, W-135, and C and A capsular polysaccharides

What is the only encapsulated fungal pathogen?

Cryptococcus

What type of spore is asexual and formed of hyphae?

Conidia

What is the only *Plasmodium* that is quartan?

Plasmodium malariae; the others are tertian.

Which bacteria are associated with the following pigment production?

    Red pigmentation

Serratia

    Black-gray pigmentation

Corynebacterium diphtheriae

    Pyocyanin (blue-green)

Pseudomonas aeruginosa

    Yellow pigmentation

Staphylococcus aureus

Which carcinoma— Burkitt's lymphoma, nasopharyngeal carcinoma, hepatocellular carcinoma, or thymic carcinoma—is *not* associated with EBV?

Hepatocellular carcinoma is associated with hepatitis B and C infections, not with EBV.

What capsular serotype is associated with *Escherichia coli*–induced meningitis?

K1 capsule

What two Ags must be positive for a patient to have chronic active hepatitis?

HB_sAg and HB_eAg

In the window phase of a hepatitis B infection, which Abs do you see?

HB_cAb and HB_eAb. You **see** the antibodies **c** and **e.**

True or false? All streptococci are catalase-negative.

True

In what trimester is the fetus most vulnerable to congenital rubella syndrome?

The first trimester

What virus causes hoof-and-mouth disease?

Vesicular stomatitis virus

Which gram-negative diplococcus grows on chocolate agar? Thayer-Martin medium?

Meningococcus grows on chocolate agar, and *Gonococcus* grows on Thayer-Martin medium.

Which protozoal parasitic vaginal infection produces a positive whiff test with KOH staining?

Trichomonas vaginalis (treat with metronidazole)

Name the *DNA virus*:

Linear dsDNA; enveloped; virion-associated polymerases; replicates in the cytoplasm

Poxvirus

Linear dsDNA; nuclear envelope; icosahedral; replicates in the nucleus

Herpes virus

Linear dsDNA; naked; replicates in the nucleus

Adenovirus

ssDNA; naked; icosahedral; replicates in the nucleus

Parvovirus

Partially dsDNA circular; enveloped; virion-associated polymerases; has RNA intermediate; replicates in the nucleus

Hepadnavirus

Circular dsDNA; naked; icosahedral; replicates in the nucleus

Papovavirus

What fungus is urease positive?

Cryptococcus

What bacterium is characterized by large boxcar-shaped gram-positive rods and is spore-forming, aerobic, and associated with cutaneous infections and woolsorter's disease?

Bacillus anthracis

Is the Salk polio vaccine inactivated?

Yes

True or false? All negative sense RNA viruses are enveloped.

True. They all have helical nucleocapsids and virion-associated polymerases too.

What urease-positive non–lactose-fermenting gram-negative rod with swarming-type motility is associated with staghorn renal calculi?

Proteus

With what two viruses are Reye's syndrome associated?

Varicella virus and influenza virus

Which organism releases endotoxins *prior* to cell death?

Neisseria meningitidis

Clue cells are associated with which organism that causes vaginal discharge?

Gardnerella vaginalis

What is the name of the bullet-shaped virus?

Rhabdovirus

What fungus is characterized by India ink staining of the CSF that produces colorless cells with a halo on a black background?

Cryptococcus neoformans

What does hepatitis D virus need from hepatitis B virus to be infective?	HB$_s$Ag as its envelope
Which type of hepatitis is a calicivirus?	Hepatitis E (enteric)
What genus is known as the smallest free living bacteria? (hint: has no cell wall and has sterols in the membrane)	*Mycoplasma*
What three organs can be affected by *Trypanosoma cruzi*?	Heart, esophagus, and colon. Remember, you get **megas:** cardio**mega**ly, **mega**esophagus, and **mega**colon.
Which serotypes of HPV are associated with plantar warts?	HPV serotypes 1 and 4
What facultative gram-negative anaerobic rod is motile, ferments lactose, and is the MCC of UTIs?	*Escherichia coli*
What is the only dsRNA virus?	Reovirus
What are the four segmented RNA viruses?	1. **B**unyavirus 2. **O**rthomyxovirus 3. **R**eovirus 4. **A**renavirus Remember **BORA.**

What type of *Plasmodium* affects

Only mature RBCs?	*Plasmodium malariae*
Only reticulocytes?	*Plasmodium vivax*
RBCs of all ages?	*Plasmodium falciparum*

What is the major cell membrane sterol found in fungi?	Ergosterol
What Ab is an indication of low transmissibility for hepatitis?	HB_eAb
What is the term for RNA-dependent DNA polymerase?	Reverse transcriptase
Which gram-positive bacteria infection of infancy is associated with ingestion of *honey*?	*Clostridium botulinum*
Which trematode is associated with *bladder carcinoma* in Egypt and Africa?	*Schistosoma haematobium*
Which encapsulated fungus is found in soil enriched with pigeon droppings?	*Cryptococcus neoformans*

What virus lies dormant in the

Trigeminal ganglia?	Herpes I
Dorsal root ganglia?	Varicella
Sensory ganglia of S2 and S3?	Herpes II
What is the name of the exotoxin *Shigella dysenteriae* produces, which interferes with the 60S ribosomal subunit and results in eukaryotic protein synthesis inhibition?	Shiga toxin (enterohemorrhagic *Escherichia coli* produces Vero toxin, which is quite similar to shiga toxin)

What protozoal parasite forms flasked-shaped lesions in the duodenum, is transmitted via fecal-oral route, and is commonly seen in campers who drank stream water?

Giardia lamblia (treat with metronidazole)

What color do fungi stain with PAS? Silver stain?

Hot pink with PAS and grey to black with silver stain

A *tropical fish* enthusiast has granulomatous lesions and cellulitis; what is the most likely offending organism?

Mycobacterium marinum

Which dimorphic fungus is found as Arthroconidia in desert sand of the southwestern United States (e.g., San Joaquin Valley)?

Coccidioides immitis

Which mycoplasma species is associated with urethritis, prostatitis, and renal calculi?

Ureaplasma urealyticum

What tick is the vector for babesiosis?

Ixodes (also the vector for Lyme disease)

What is the only DNA virus that does not replicate its DNA in the nucleus of the host cell?

Poxvirus replicates its DNA in the cytoplasm.

What organism would you suspect in a patient with diarrhea after eating rice?

Bacillus cereus

What small gram-negative facultative intracellular rod is transmitted to human host by *Dermacentor* tick bite?

Francisella tularensis

True or false? Cestodes have no GI tract.	True. They absorb nutrients from the host's GI tract.
What negative sense RNA virus is associated with parotitis, pancreatitis, and orchitis?	Mumps

What is the size of a *positive* PPD test for the following? (Reactive)

IV drug abuser	> 10 mm
Patient with AIDS	> 5 mm
Recent immigrant from India	> 10 mm
Healthy suburban male without any medical illnesses	> 15 mm
Posttransplantation patient taking immunosuppressive agents	> 5 mm
What are the only two picornaviruses that do *not* lead to aseptic meningitis?	Rhinovirus and hepatitis A virus
Which cestode in raw or rare *beef* containing cysticerci results in intestinal tapeworms?	*Taenia saginata*
What DNA viral disease is associated with aplastic crisis in patients with sickle cell anemia?	Parvovirus B-19
What glycoprotein in the HIV virus attaches to CD4?	GP120

What Enterobacteriaceae are prone to produce osteomyelitis in sickle cell patients?	*Salmonella*
What organism is commonly associated with a cellulitis from an *animal bite*?	*Pasteurella multocida*
What fungus is seen as colored cauliflower lesions?	Chromomycosis
What is the reservoir for the togavirus?	Birds
What are the two exceptions to the rule "all cocci are gram positive"?	Both *Neisseria* and *Moraxella* are gram-negative cocci.
What nematode is known as *hookworms*? What is the treatment?	*Necator americanus* is treated with mebendazole and iron therapy.
What HIV structural gene produces GP120 and GP41?	*env* structural protein
Which hemoflagellate species causes *kala azar*?	*Leishmania donovani* (kala azar is also known as visceral leishmaniasis)
What DNA virus is associated with heterophile-negative mononucleosis?	CMV; remember, EBV is associated with heterophile-positive mononucleosis.
What negative sense RNA virus is associated with intracytoplasmic inclusion bodies called Negri bodies?	Rabies
What large, spore-forming, gram-positive anaerobic rod is associated with infections due to puncture wounds and trauma?	*Clostridium tetani*

What is the vector for Chagas disease?

The reduviid bug

What is the polarity (i.e., 5′-3′ or 3′-5′) of a positive sense RNA?

Positive sense RNA means it can serve as mRNA and therefore has **5′-3′ polarity**.

What viral infection is associated with black vomit?

Yellow fever (flavivirus)

What encapsulated gram-negative, lactose-fermenting rod is associated with pneumonia in patients with alcoholism, diabetes, and chronic lung disease?

Klebsiella pneumoniae

What is the essential reservoir host for *Toxoplasma gondii*?

The cat

What gram-positive anaerobic rod with branching filaments is a component of the normal flora of the mouth and female genital tract and is responsible for draining abscesses with sulfur granules in the exudates?

Actinomyces israelii

What is the term for *Candida* infection of the oral mucosa?

Thrush

What is the term for fungi that can convert from hyphal to yeast forms?

Dimorphic

To what viral family does the polio virus belong?

Picornaviridae

Name at least three bacteria that use capsules to prevent immediate destruction from the host's defense system.

Streptococcus pneumoniae, Klebsiella pneumoniae, Haemophilus influenzae, Pseudomonas aeruginosa, and *Neisseria meningitidis;* also *Cryptococcus neoformans,* a fungus

True or false? There are no persistent infections with naked viruses?

True. They lyse the host cell

What virus is associated with progressive multifocal leukoencephalopathy?

JC virus

What bacterium is a gram-negative, oxidase-positive aerobic rod that produces a grapelike odor and pyocyanin pigmentation?

Pseudomonas aeruginosa

Which three organisms cause heterophilic negative mononucleosis?

CMV, *Toxoplasma gondii,* and *Listeria*

What bacterium found in poorly preserved canned food causes flaccid paralysis?

Clostridium botulinum

Which two negative sense RNA viruses have neuraminidase enzymes?

Mumps and influenza virus

What *Staphylococcus aureus* protein inhibits phagocytosis?

Protein A

Which four bacteria require cysteine for growth?

Pasteurella, Brucella, Legionella, and *Francisella* (all of the -ellas)

What fungus causes endocarditis in IV drug users?

Candida albicans

What viruses are associated with Cowdry type A intranuclear inclusions?

Herpes virus I and II

Which streptococcal species is associated with dental caries and infective endocarditis in patients with poor oral hygiene?

Streptococcus viridans

What is the term for cestode-encysted larvae found in intermediate hosts?

Cysticerci

What fungus is characterized by hypopigmented spots on the thorax, spaghetti-and-meatball KOH staining, and pityriasis or tinea versicolor?

Malassezia furfur (treat with selenium sulfide)

What nematode is known as *threadworms*? What is the treatment?

Strongyloides stercoralis is treated with thiabendazole.

What are known as jumping genes?

Transposons

What virus produces koilocytic cells on a Papanicolaou (Pap) smear?

HPV

Which dimorphic fungus is endemic in the Ohio, Mississippi, Missouri, and Eastern Great Lakes, is found in soil with bird and bat feces, and is associated with infections in spelunkers and chicken coop cleaners?

Histoplasma capsulatum

Which of the following Enterobacteriaceae family members—*Yersinia*, *Klebsiella*, *Enterobacter*, *Escherichia*, *Proteus*, and *Citrobacter*—do *not* ferment lactose?

All are lactose fermenters except *Yersinia* and *Proteus*.

What two HIV regulatory genes down-regulate MHC class I expression in the host?

nef and *tat* genes

What size ribosomes do fungi have?

80S ribosomes (because they are eukaryotic)

IMMUNOLOGY

What test is done to diagnose CGD?

Nitroblue tetrazolium reduction test (NBT). It is negative in patients with CGD because there is no production of oxygen radicals.

What is the valence of an Ig molecule equal to?

The number of Ags that the Ab can bind

What is the name of the process that ensures that each B cell produces only one heavy-chain variable domain and one light chain?

Allelic exclusion. It is to ensure that one B cell produces only one Ab.

What is the major Ab of the primary immune response?

IgM

What form of immunity is responsible for removal of *intracellular infections*?

Cell-mediated immunity

True or false? *Direct* fluorescent Ab test is used to detect Abs in a patient?

False. **Direct** tests detect *Ags;* **indirect** tests detect *Abs.*

What is the triad of Wiskott-Aldrich syndrome?

Thrombocytopenia, eczema, and immunodeficiency is the triad of this **X-linked recessive** disorder.

What complement factor deficiency leads to

    Increased susceptibility to pyogenic infections?

C3 deficiency

    Recurrent gonococcal infections?

C5-C8 deficiency

    Leukocyte adhesion deficiency with poor opsonization?

C1, C2, or C4 deficiency

    Hereditary angioedema?

C1 inhibitor (C1-INH)

Which IgG cannot activate complement?

IgG4

Name the T-cell CD marker:

    Essential for Ab isotype switching (for B cell binding)

CD40 ligand

    Interacts with MHC class I molecules

CD8

    Expressed on all T cells and is needed as a signal transducer for the T cell receptor

CD3

    Interacts with MHC class II molecules

CD4

    Is a costimulatory molecule in T cell activation

CD28

What three cells are essential for T-cell differentiation in the thymus?

Dendritic cells, macrophages, and thymic epithelial cells

What is the only specific Ag-presenting cell?

B cells; macrophages and dendritic cells are nonspecific.

What is the tetrad of Jarisch-Herxheimer reaction?

Rigors, leukopenia, decrease in blood pressure, and increase in temperature

What is the name of the B cell that secretes Ig?

Plasma cell (mature B lymphocyte)

What would be the result if an Ab were cleaved with papain?

There would be two Fab and Fc regions.

What is the bone marrow maturation time for a phagocytic cell?

14 days

Which leukotrienes are associated with the late-phase inflammatory response?

LTC_4 and LTD_4

What is the term for the strength of the association between Ag and an Ab?

Affinity (**one** of each)

True or false? More Ag is needed to produce a secondary immune response than a first immune response.

False. **Fewer** Ags are needed to trigger a secondary response.

What is the term for the strength of association between multiple Ab-binding sites and multiple antigenic determinants?

Avidity (more than one binding site)

What Ig mediates ADCC via K cells, opsonizes, and is the Ig of the secondary immune response?

IgG

What test is used to detect anti-RBC Abs seen in hemolytic anemia?

Coombs test

What subset of T cells recognizes the MHC class I Ags?

CD8+ T cells (cytotoxic)
Remember, $8 \times 1 = 8$ (CD**8** $\times$ MHC class **I** = **8**); $4 \times 2 =$ 8 (CD**4** $\times$ MHC class **II** = **8**)

What cell surface marker is found on activated helper T cells?

CD40

What are the five Ig isotypes?

IgA, IgD, IgE, IgG, and IgM

Which integrin mediates the adhesion to endothelial cells for migration in and out of the blood during an immune response?

β_2-integrins

What type of hypersensitivity is an Ab-mediated response against our own cells, receptors, or membranes via IgG or IgM?

Type II hypersensitivity reaction

What is the term to describe the limited portion of an Ag that is recognized by an Ab?

Antigenic determinant (epitope)

What cytokine do Th1 cells secrete to inhibit Th2 cell function?

INF-γ

What three cells are essential for T-cell maturation?

Thymic epithelial cells, dendritic cells, and macrophages

What is the term for a single isolated antigenic determinant?

Hapten (not immunogenic)

What are the two opsonizing factors?

The Fc region of IgG and C3b

What is the most common Ig deficiency?

IgA deficiency; patients commonly present with recurrent sinopulmonary infections and GI disturbances.

What is the name of the B cell–rich area of the spleen?

Primary follicle (in the white pulp)

What IL, produced by macrophages, is chemotactic for neutrophils?

IL-8. It not only is chemotactic, it also acts as an adhesive for neutrophils.

What Ig prevents bacterial adherence to mucosal surfaces?

IgA

What are the three rules of clonal selection?

1. One cell type
2. One Ab type
3. Random selection of hypervariable regions, and only cells with bound Ag undergo clonal expansion

What is a plasma cell's life expectancy?

7 to 14 days

What are defined by Ag-binding specificity?

Idiotypes

What type of binding occurs with one Fab or one idiotype of IgG?

Affinity

What molecule that is needed to trigger T cell activation is noncovalently linked to TCR?

CD3 molecule. It transmits signals to the inside of the T cell to trigger activation.

What is the term for Ags that activate B cells without T-cell signaling?

Thymus-independent Ags

What are the three rules governing a secondary immune response?

1. **Covalent** bonding between the hapten and carrier
2. B-cell exposure to **hapten twice**
3. T-cell exposure to **carrier twice**

What type of hypersensitivity is a T cell-mediated response to Ags that are *not* activated by Ab or complement?

Type IV hypersensitivity reaction (delayed type because of the 48–96 hour latency)

Name the macrophages by location:

Liver

Kupffer cells

Lungs

Alveolar macrophages

CNS

Microglial cells

Kidney

Mesangial macrophages

What is the first human disease successfully treated with gene therapy?

Adenosine deaminase (ADA) deficiency

What receptors are the best markers for NK cells?

CD16 and CD56

True or false? Ag-Ab binding is irreversible.

False. It is reversible because the Ags and Abs are linked covalently.

What three major cell lines participate in the acquired immune system?

T cells, B cells, and macrophages

What test is used to screen for HIV?	ELISA. It detects anti-p24 IgG.
During what stage of B-cell development is IgM first seen on the surface?	Immature B cells
What Ig is responsible for ADCC of parasites, has a high-affinity Fc receptor on mast cells and basophils, and is responsible for the allergic response?	IgE
True or false? B-cell Ag receptors can be secreted.	True. B cell antigen receptors are Abs.
Are more Abs produced in a primary or a secondary immune response?	More Ab is produced in less time in a **secondary** immune response (shorter lag period).
By which process do Abs make microorganisms more easily ingested via phagocytosis?	Opsonization
What MHC class acts to remove *foreign* Ags from the body?	MHC class II Ags. This is accomplished via CD4 T cells.
What disorder is characterized by autoantibodies to IF?	Pernicious anemia
What cytokines do Th2 cells secrete to inhibit Th1 cell function?	IL-4, IL-10, and IL-13
What is the term for the number of Ag-binding sites on an Ig?	Valence

Which major cell type is found in the red pulp of the spleen?	RBCs. That is why it is called red pulp.
What is the name of the pathway that produces leukotrienes?	Lipoxygenase pathway, from arachidonic acid
What is the term to describe basophils that have left the bloodstream and entered a tissue?	Mast cells
What are the three major functions of secretory IgA?	1. IgA receptor 2. Transport of IgA across epithelial barriers 3. Protection of IgA from degradative proteases
What IL is important in myeloid cell development?	IL-3 (**3** face down is an **M**)
What is the term for different classes and subclasses of the same gene products?	Isotypes
What is the first Ab a baby makes?	IgM
What test, by using specific Abs to different receptors, allows for rapid analysis of cell types in a blood sample?	Flow cytometric analysis
What is the name of the T cell–rich area of the spleen?	PALS
What three complement fragments are also anaphylatoxins?	C3a, C4a, and C5a

Name the B-cell CD marker:

Required for class switching signals from T cells	CD40
Receptor for EBV	CD21; it is a complement receptor for cleaved C3
Used clinically to count B cells in blood	CD19

What immunologic test checks for a reaction between Abs and a particular Ag? (hint: ABO typing)

Agglutination test

Which leukotriene is chemotactic for neutrophils?

LTB_4

What Ig is associated with mucosal surfaces and external secretions?

IgA

What are the genetic variants of a molecule within members of the same species?

Allotypes

What cytokine do CD4 T cells secrete to activate B cells when the specific peptide in the groove of the MHC II molecule interacts with the TCR?

IL-4 is secreted to activate B cells. This begins the second step in the immune response, known as **Activation**. CD4 T cells to activate macrophages secrete INF-α.

Which protein prevents internal binding of self proteins within an MHC class II cell?

Invariant chain

What would be the result if an Ab were cleaved with pepsin?

There would be a Fab' region; thus, it would still be able to participate in precipitation and agglutination.

Why are patients with CGD *not* prone to develop infections from catalase-negative bacteria?

Catalase-negative bacteria secrete H_2O_2 as a byproduct (remember, catalase breaks down H_2O_2), allowing the neutrophils to use it as the substrate for the other toxic metabolites. Patients with CGD are prone to catalase-positive bacterial infections.

What are the two chains of the TCR that are mainly found on the skin and mucosal surfaces?

γ- and δ-chains

Which IL is associated with increases of IgG and IgE?

IL-4

What branch of the immune system is acquired in response to an Ag?

Adaptive branch. The adaptive branch of the immune system has a slow initiation with rapid responses thereafter.

True or false? T cells can recognize, bind, and internalize *unprocessed* Ags.

False. B cells recognize **unprocessed** Ags, but T cells can recognize *only* **processed** Ags.

What type of hypersensitivity is a result of high circulating levels of soluble *immune complexes* made up of IgG or IgM Abs?

Type III hypersensitivity reaction

At what stage of B-cell development can IgM or IgD be expressed on the cell surface?

Mature B cell; the memory B cell can have IgG, IgA, or IgE on its surface.

What T cell deficiency syndrome is associated with facial anomalies, hypoparathyroidism, thymic hypoplasia, and recurrent viral and fungal infections?

DiGeorge syndrome, which is due to a failure of the third and fourth pharyngeal pouch development. Remember, B cell deficiencies are associated with **extracellular** infection. T cell deficiencies are associated with **intracellular** infections.

What is the stimulus for the classical pathway activation?

Ag-Ab complexes. The alternative pathway protects without use of Abs; the pathogen is the stimulus.

What is the first membrane-bound Ig on B cell membranes?

IgM; IgD follows shortly thereafter.

What region of the Ig does not change with class switching?

Hypervariable region

In MHC class II molecules, what chain blocks access to the peptide-binding groove during transportation within the cell, ensuring that the MHC class II–peptide *complex* is transported to the surface?

Invariant chain. This is essential because the CD4 T cells have antigen receptors **only** for peptides bound to the MHC II molecule. (MHC restriction)

What chromosome codes for HLA gene products?

The short arm of **chromosome 6**

What cells are atypical on a peripheral blood smear in heterophil-positive mononucleosis?

T cells, not B cells

What is the major Ig of the secondary immune response in the mucosal barriers?

IgA

What *AR* disorder is seen by age 1 to 2 with recurrent sinopulmonary infections, uncoordinated muscle movements, and dilation of the blood vessels?

Ataxia-telangiectasia

What are the four chemotactic agents?

1. C5a
2. Leukotriene B_4
3. IL-8
4. Bacterial peptides

What subset of CD4 helper T cells stimulate B-cell division and differentiation?

Th2

Which region of the variable domain comprises the Ag-binding site of the Ab?

Hypervariable region (three per light chain; three per heavy chain)

True or false? The increased oxygen consumption after phagocytosis is for ATP production.

False; it is for the production of toxic metabolites.

What is the limited portion of a large Ag that will actually be recognized and bound to an Ab and that contains approximately five to six amino acids or four to five hexose units?

Antigenic determinant (epitope). (Idiotypes bind to epitopes.)

What complement factor or factors are associated with

Chemotaxis?

C5a

Membrane attack complex (MAC)?

C5–C9

Opsonization?	C3b
Anaphylaxis?	C3a, C4a, C5a
What happens to the Ab specificity when class switching occurs in mature B cells?	As the isotype is switched, the Ab specificity does **not** change because it does not affect the variable chains.
What IL down-regulates cell mediated immunity?	IL-10

Name the type of graft described by these transplants:

From one site to another on the same person	**Auto**graft
Between genetically identical individuals	**Iso**graft
From one person to the next (the same species)	**Allo**graft
From one species to another	**Xeno**graft
What is the name of the process in which cells migrate toward an attractant along a concentration gradient?	Chemotaxis
What are the two functions of the thymus in T-cell differentiation?	Hormone secretion for T-cell differentiation and T-cell education to recognize self from nonself

What is the name of the T cell–rich area of the lymph node?

Paracortex

What cell surface marker do all T cells have?

CD3

True or false? Patients with common variable hypogammaglobinemia have B cells in the peripheral blood.

True. Common variable hypogammaglobinemia first appears by the time patients reach their 20s and is associated with a gradual decrease in Ig levels over time.

What is the Ig associated with the primary immune response?

IgM

What MHC class of antigens do all nucleated cells carry on their surface membranes?

MHC class I antigens; they are also found on the surface of platelets.

What Ig is responsible for activation of complement, opsonization, and ADCC and is actively transported across the placenta?

IgG

What type of Ag do T cells recognize?

Processed antigenic peptides bound in the groove of the MHC molecule

What Ig is the major protective factor in colostrum?

IgA

What is the second cell involved in the immune response?

The CD4 T cell; the APC is the first cell in the immune response.

What is the term for thymic induction of T cells with *high*-affinity Ag receptors for *self* that are programmed to undergo apoptosis?

Negative selection. This helps to prevent autoimmune diseases.

What five main oxidizing reactions are used to kill ingested organisms?

1. H_2O_2
2. Superoxide
3. Hydroxyl radical
4. Myeloperoxidase
5. Hypochlorous acid

What Ig is associated with ADCC for parasite?

IgE

True or false? RBCs do *not* have MHC class I Ags on their surface.

True. Remember, all *nucleated cells* (and platelets) have MHC class I Ags, and RBCs are not nucleated.

What Ig is associated with mast cell and basophil binding?

IgE. It attaches via receptor for the Fc region of the heavy epsilon chain.

What IL do T cells secrete to induce T- and B-cell division?

IL-2. T cells express IL-2 receptors on their surface to induce self-expression.

Development of what T cell line follows *low* affinity for self-MHC class II Ags in the thymus?

CD4+ T cells

What is the term for a substance secreted by a leukocyte in response to a stimulus?

Cytokine. If a cytokine affects another class of leukocytes, it is called an **interleukin**.

What subset of CD4 T cells is responsible for mast cell and eosinophil precursor proliferation?

Th2 cells

What are the four major functions of the acquired immune system?

1. Recognize self from nonself
2. Amplify via cell division or complementation
3. Control the level of the response
4. Remove foreign material

What endotoxin receptor is the best marker for macrophages?

CD14

What is the term for the inherent ability to induce a specific immune response?

Immunogenicity; antigenicity refers to Ab/lymphocyte reaction to a specific substance.

What molecule differentiates the MHC class I from II Ag? (Hint: it's in the light chain.)

The β_2-microglobin. It is the separately encoded β-chain for class I Ags.

What B cell disorder is characterized by pre-B cells in the bone marrow, no circulating B cells in plasma, normal cell-mediated immunity, low Igs, and appearance by 6 months of age?

Bruton X-linked hypogammaglobinemia. Tyrosine kinase deficiency leads to inadequate B cell maturation.

What subtype of IgG does *not* bind to staphylococcal A protein?

IgG3

What mast cell mediator is a chemotactic agent?

Eosinophil chemotactic factor A

What is the major Ig of the secondary immune response?

IgG

What T-cell surface projection recognizes and reacts to foreign Ags (presented by APCs)?

TCR

What is the confirmatory test for HIV?

Western blot

What is the name of the major chemotactic agent released from

    Neutrophils?

Leukotriene B4 (LTB4)

    Macrophages?

IL-8 (IL-1 and TNF-γ also)

The blood serum? (Hint: it is a complement factor.)	C5a
Bacteria?	F-Met-Peptides
What cell surface marker is found on blood B cells?	CD19
What is the name of the B cell–rich area in the lymph node?	Primary follicle of the cortex
What are the four ways to down-regulate the immune system?	1. Decrease concentrations of Ag levels 2. Administer IgG in high concentrations 3. Inhibit B cells with Ag bound to IgG (complexes) 4. Turn off the original T or B cell with anti-Ab
What is the only Ig that crosses the placenta?	IgG
What is given to pregnant women within 24 hours after birth to eliminate Rh+ fetal blood cells from their circulation?	Rh_o (D) immune globulin (RhoGAM), an anti-RhD IgG antibody, prevents generation of RhD-specific memory B cells in the mother.
What IL is essential for lymphoid cell development?	IL-7 (A **7** upside down is an **L**; **L** is for **L**ymphoid)
What type of cell can never leave the lymph node?	Plasma cell
Via what pathway is glycolysis increased after phagocytosis?	HMP shunt
What is the term for a delay in the onset of normal IgG synthesis seen in the fifth to sixth month of life?	Transient hypogammaglobinemia of infancy; it usually resolves by age 16 to 30 months.

What subset of CD4 helper T-cell function is helping the development of CD8 T cells?

Th1; they are also responsible for delayed-type hypersensitivity (type IV)

What is the term for the strength of the association between Ags and Abs?

Avidity. There is a positive correlation between valence numbers and avidity.

What type of Ag do B cells recognize?

Free, unprocessed Ag

What Ig is associated with Ag recognition receptor on the surface of mature B cells?

IgD; IgM is also correct.

Which chromosome is associated with MHC genes?

Chromosome 6

What is the term for processing an APC's pinocytosed material by fusing with a lysosomal granule and cleaving the Ag into peptide fragments?

Ag processing; it is needed for class I molecules. Class II molecules have an invariant chain that protects them from breakdown.

What is the most common precipitin test used in clinical medicine?

Radial **I**mmuno**D**iffusion (**RID**) for Ig levels.

What Ig activates the complement cascade most efficiently?

IgM

What assay is used to identify MHC class I molecules?

Microcytotoxic assay

Which IL increases IgA synthesis?

IL-5. It also stimulates eosinophil proliferation.

What is the term for an immunogenic agent that is too small to elicit an immune response?	Hapten; if it is coupled with a carrier, it may become immunogenic.

What type II hypersensitivity disorder is defined as

Autoantibodies directed against ACh receptors?	Myasthenia gravis
Autoantibodies directed against platelet integrin?	Autoimmune thrombocytopenia purpura
Autoantibodies against the type IV collagen in the basement membrane of the kidneys and lungs?	Goodpasture syndrome
Autoantibodies directed against the TSH receptor?	Graves disease
Autoantibodies directed against RBC Ag I?	Autoimmune hemolytic anemia

What Ig activates the alternate pathway, neutralizes bacterial endotoxins and viruses, and prevents bacterial adherence?	IgA
What enzyme is deficient in patients with CGD?	NADPH oxidase is deficient, resulting in an inability to produce toxic metabolites.
What subtype of IgG does *not* activate complement cascade?	IgG4
What two cell lines of the immune system do *not* belong to the innate branch?	T and B-cells belong to the *adaptive* branch, whereas PMNs, NK cells, eosinophils, macrophages, and monocytes belong to the *innate* branch.

What subset of T cells recognizes the MHC class II Ags?

CD4+ T cells (helper)

What T cell line arises from *low* affinity for self-MHC class I Ags in the thymus?

CD8+ T cells

What MHC class functions as a *target* for elimination of *abnormal host cells*?

MHC class I Ags (the endogenous pathway). This allows the body to eliminate tumor cells, virus-infected cells—anything the body recognizes as nonself via CD8+ T cells.

What are the three polymorphonuclear leukocytes? Be specific.

Neutrophils, eosinophils, and basophils

5 _____ Physiology

In a ventricular pacemaker cell, what phase of the action potential is affected by NE?

Phase 4; NE increases the slope of the prepotential, allowing threshold to be reached sooner, and increases the rate of firing.

Anatomical and alveolar dead spaces together constitute what space?

Physiologic dead space is the *total dead space* of the respiratory system.

What three organs are necessary for the production of vitamin D_3 (cholecalciferol)?

Skin, liver, and kidneys

What is the effect of LH on the production of adrenal androgens?

LH has **no effect** on the production of adrenal androgens; ACTH stimulates adrenal androgen production.

What four conditions result in secondary hyperaldosteronism?

1. CHF
2. Vena caval obstruction or constriction
3. Hepatic cirrhosis
4. Renal artery stenosis

What are the five hormones produced by *Sertoli* cells?

1. Inhibin
2. Estradiol (E_2)
3. Androgen-binding protein
4. Meiosis inhibiting factor (in fetal tissue)
5. Antimüullerian hormone

What is the term for the negative resting membrane potential moving *toward threshold*?

Depolarization (i.e., Na^+ influx)

Does the left or right vagus nerve innervate the SA node?

Right vagus innervates the **SA node** and the **left** vagus innervates the **AV node**

How does ventricular *repolarization* take place, base to apex or vice versa?

Repolarization is from base to apex and from epicardium to endocardium.

What is the term for any region of the respiratory system that is *incapable of gas exchange*?

Anatomical dead space, which ends at the level of the terminal bronchioles.

What four factors shift the Hgb-O$_2$ dissociation curve to the right? What is the consequence of this shift?

Increased CO$_2$, H$^+$, temperature, and 2,3-BPG levels all shift the curve to the right, thereby making the O$_2$ easier to remove (decreased affinity) from the Hgb molecule.

What two factors result in the *apex* of the lung being *hypoperfused*?

Decreased pulmonary arterial pressure (low perfusion) and less-distensible vessels (high resistance) result in decreased blood flow at the apex.

What is the ratio of pulmonary to systemic blood flow?

1:1. Remember, the flow through the pulmonary circuit and the systemic circuit are equal.

To differentiate central from nephrogenic diabetes insipidus, after an injection of ADH, which will show a decreased urine flow?

Central. Remember, there is a deficiency in ADH production in the central form.

In what area of the GI tract are water-soluble vitamins absorbed?

Duodenum

What wave is the cause of the following venous pulse deflections?

The rise in right atrial pressure secondary to blood filling and terminating when the tricuspid valves opens

V wave

The bulging of the tricuspid valve into the right atrium	C wave
The contraction of the right atrium	A wave

What are the four functions of saliva?
1. Provide antibacterial action
2. Lubricate
3. Begin CHO digestion
4. Begin fat digestion

When a person goes from supine to standing, what happens to the following?

Dependent venous pressure	Increases
Dependent venous blood volume	Increases
Cardiac output	Decreases
BP	Decreases
	Remember, the **carotid sinus reflex** attempts to **compensate** by **increasing** both **TPR** and **heart rate.**

When does the hydrostatic pressure in Bowman's capsule play a role in opposing filtration?

It normally does not play a role in filtration but becomes important when there is an **obstruction downstream.**

What happens to intrapleural pressure when the diaphragm is contracted during inspiration?

Intrapleural pressure decreases (becomes more negative).

What is used as an index of cortisol secretion?

Urinary 17-OH steroids

If the *pH is low* with *increased CO_2* levels and *decreased HCO_3^-* levels, what is the acid-base disturbance?

Combined metabolic and respiratory acidosis

What is the term that refers to the number of *channels open* in a cell membrane?

Membrane conductance (think conductance = channels open)

What are the five tissues in which glucose uptake is insulin independent?

1. CNS
2. Renal tubules
3. β Islet cells of the pancreas
4. RBCs
5. GI mucosa

Place in order from fastest to slowest the rate of gastric emptying for CHO, fat, liquids, and proteins.

Liquids, CHO, protein, fat

Is most of the coronary artery blood flow during systole or diastole?

Diastole. During systole the left ventricle contracts, resulting in intramyocardial vessel compression and therefore very little blood flow in the coronary circulation.

What modified smooth muscle cells of the kidney monitor BP in the afferent arteriole?

The JG cells

What are the three functions of surfactant?

1. Increase compliance
2. Decrease surface tension
3. Decrease probability of pulmonary edema formation

Name the hormone— glucagon, insulin, or epinephrine:

  Glycogenolytic, gluconeogenic, lipolytic, glycolytic, and stimulated by hypoglycemia

Epinephrine

Glycogenolytic, gluconeogenic, lipolytic, glycolytic, proteolytic, and stimulated by hypoglycemia and AAs	Glucagon
Glycogenic, gluconeogenic, lipogenic, proteogenic, glycolytic, and stimulated by hyperglycemia, AAs, fatty acids, ketosis, ACh, GH, and β-agonists	Insulin
Is the hydrophobic or hydrophilic end of the phospholipids of the cell membrane facing the *aqueous environment*?	**Hydrophobic** (water-insoluble) end faces the aqueous environment and the hydrophilic (water-soluble) end faces the interior of the cell.
What type of muscle is characterized by no myoglobin, anaerobic glycolysis, high ATPase activity, and large muscle mass?	White muscle; short term too
What percentage of CO_2 is carried in the plasma as HCO_3^-?	**90%** as HCO_3^-, **5%** as **carbamino** compounds, and **5%** as **dissolved CO_2**
What is the most potent male sex hormone?	Dihydrotestosterone
With a decrease in arterial diastolic pressure, what happens to	
Stroke volume?	Decreases
TPR?	Decreases
Heart rate?	Decreases

What linkage of complex CHOs does pancreatic amylase hydrolyze? What three complexes are formed?

Amylase hydrolyzes **α-1,4-glucoside** linkages, forming **α-limit dextrins, maltotriose,** and **maltose.**

Does the heart rate determine the diastolic or systolic interval?

Heart rate determines the **diastolic** interval, and **contractility** determines the **systolic** interval.

On a graphical representation of filtration, reabsorption, and excretion, when does glucose first appear in the urine?

At the **beginning of splay** is when the renal threshold for glucose occurs and the excess begins to spill over into the urine.

What is the relationship between preload and the passive tension in a muscle?

They are **directly** related; the **greater** the preload, the **greater** the passive tension in the muscle and the **greater** the prestretch of a sarcomere.

What is the *rate-limiting step* in the synthetic pathway of *NE* at the *adrenergic nerve* terminal?

The **conversion** of **tyrosine to dopamine** in the **cytoplasm**

How many days *prior to* ovulation does *LH* surge occur in the menstrual cycle?

1 day prior to ovulation

How are flow through the loop of Henle and concentration of urine related?

As **flow increases,** the **urine** becomes more **dilute** because of decreased time for H_2O reabsorption.

What is the Po_2 of aortic blood in fetal circulation?

60%

How do elevated blood glucose levels decrease GH secretion? (Hint: what inhibitory hypothalamic hormone is stimulated by IGF-1?)

Somatotrophins are stimulated by IGF-1, and they **inhibit** GH secretion. **GHRH stimulates** GH secretion.

What segment of the nephron has the highest concentration of inulin? Lowest concentration of inulin?

Terminal collecting duct has the **highest** concentration and **Bowman's capsule** has the **lowest** concentration of inulin.

What type of resistance system, high or low, is formed when resistors are added in a *series*?

A **high-resistance** system is formed when resistors are added in a series.

What hormones, secreted in proportion to the size of the *placenta*, are an index of fetal well-being?

hCS and serum **estriol,** which are produced by the fetal liver and placenta, respectively, are used as estimates of **fetal** well-being.

What primary acid-base disturbance is caused by an *increase in alveolar ventilation* (decreasing CO_2 levels) resulting in the reaction *shifting to the left* and *decreasing both H^+ and HCO_3^-* levels?

Respiratory **alk**alosis (summary: **low CO_2, low H^+, slightly low HCO_3^-**)

What respiratory center in the caudal pons is the center for rhythm promoting prolonged inspirations?

Apneustic center (deep breathing place)

What area of the GI tract has the highest activity of brush border enzymes?

Jejunum (upper)

What is the term to describe the increased rate of secretion of *adrenal* androgens at the onset of puberty?

Adrenarche

What period is described when a larger-than-normal stimulus is needed to produce an action potential?

Relative refractory period

Does T_3 or T_4 have a greater affinity for its *nuclear receptor*?	T_3 has a greater affinity for the **nuclear receptor** and therefore is considered the *active form.*

What are the three main functions of surfactant?

1. Lowers surface tension, so it **decreases recoil** and **increases compliance**
2. Reduces capillary filtration
3. Promotes stability in small alveoli by lowering surface tension

What is the only important physiological signal regulating the release of PTH?

Low interstitial free Ca^{2+} concentrations

What endocrine abnormality is characterized by the following changes in PTH, Ca^{2+}, and inorganic phosphate (Pi)?

PTH decreased, Ca^{2+} increased, Pi increased

Secondary **hypo**parathyroidism (vitamin D toxicity)

PTH increased, Ca^{2+} decreased, Pi decreased

Secondary **hyper**parathyroidism (vitamin D deficiency, renal disease)

PTH decreased, Ca^{2+} decreased, Pi increased

Primary **hypo**parathyroidism

PTH increased, Ca^{2+} increased, Pi decreased

Primary **hyper**parathyroidism

What is the amount in liters and percent body weight for the following compartments?

ECF

14 L, 33% of body weight

Interstitial fluid

9.3 L, 15% of body weight

ICF

28 L, 40% of body weight

Vascular fluid	4.7 L, 5% of body weight
Total body water	42 L, 67% of body weight
What hormone is secreted by the placenta late in pregnancy, stimulates mammary growth during pregnancy, mobilizes energy stores from the mother so that the fetus can use them, and has an amino acid sequence like GH?	Human chorionic somatomammotropin (hCS) or human placental lactogen (hPL)

What thyroid abnormality has the following?

TRH decreased, TSH decreased, T_4 increased	Graves disease (Increased T_4 decreases TRH and TSH through negative feedback.)
TRH increased, TSH decreased, T_4 decreased	**Secondary hypo**thyroidism/pituitary (Low TSH results in low T_4 and increased TRH because of lack of a negative feedback loop.)
TRH decreased, TSH decreased, T_4 decreased	**Tertiary hypo**thyroidism/hypothalamic (Low TRH causes all the rest to be decreased because of decreased stimulation.)
TRH increased, TSH increased, T_4 decreased	**Primary hypo**thyroidism (Low T_4 has a decreased negative feedback loop, resulting in both the hypothalamus and the anterior pituitary gland to increase TRH and TSH release, respectively.)
TRH decreased, TSH decreased, T_4 increased	**Secondary hyper**thyroidism (Increased TSH results in increased T_4 production and increased negative feedback on to hypothalamus and decreased release of TRH.)

What two stress hormones are under the permissive action of cortisol?	Glucagon and epinephrine
If the radius of a vessel *doubles*, what happens to resistance?	The resistance will **decrease** one-sixteenth of the original resistance.
What prevents the down-regulation of the receptors on the *gonadotrophs* of the anterior pituitary gland?	The **pulsatile** release of GnRH
True or false? Epinephrine has *proteolytic* metabolic effects.	False. It has **glycogenolytic** and **lipolytic** actions but not proteolytic.
What is the only 17-hydroxysteroid with hormonal activity?	Cortisol, a 21-carbon steroid, has a $-OH$ group at position 17.
Does the oncotic pressure of plasma promote filtration or reabsorption?	The oncotic pressure of plasma promotes **reabsorption** and is directly **proportional** to the filtration fraction.
Why is the base of the lung hyperventilated when a person is standing upright?	The alveoli at the base are small and very compliant, so there is a large change in their size and volume and therefore a high level of alveolar ventilation.
By removing Na^+ from the renal tubule and pumping it back into the ECF compartment, what does aldosterone do to the body's acid-base stores?	The removal of Na^+ results in the renal tubule becoming negatively charged. The negative luminal charge attracts both K^+ and H^+ into the renal tubule and promotes HCO_3^- to enter the ECF and results in **hypokalemic alkalosis**.
What hormone causes contractions of smooth muscle, regulates interdigestive motility, and prepares the intestine for the next meal?	Motilin

What two vessels in fetal circulation have the highest PO_2 levels?	Umbilical vein and ductus venosus (80%)
How many days prior to ovulation does *estradiol* peak in the menstrual cycle?	2 days prior to ovulation
What serves as a marker of *endogenous* insulin secretion?	C-peptide levels
What is the term for the total volume of air moved in and out of the respiratory system per minute?	Total ventilation (minute ventilation or minute volume)
What is the renal compensation mechanism for alkalosis?	Increase in urinary excretion of HCO^{3-}, **shifting the reaction to the right** and **increasing H^+**
What is a sign of a Sertoli cell tumor in a man?	Excess estradiol in the blood
In the systemic circulation, what blood vessels have the largest pressure drop? Smallest pressure drop?	**Arterioles** have the **largest** drop, whereas the **vena cava** has the **smallest** pressure drop in systemic circulation.
What is the major stimulus for cell division in chondroblasts?	IGF-1
What are two causes of diffusion impairment in the lungs?	Decrease in surface area and increase in membrane thickness ($Palvo_2 > Pao_2$)
What are the four effects of suckling on the mother?	1. Increased synthesis and secretion of oxytocin 2. Increased release of PIF by the hypothalamus

3. Inhibition of GnRH (suppressing FSH/LH)
4. Milk secretion

A migrating myoelectric complex is a propulsive movement of undigested material from the stomach to the small intestine to the colon. During a fast, what is the time interval of its repeats?

It repeats **every 90 to 120 minutes** and correlates with elevated levels of **motilin**.

With an *increase* in arterial systolic pressure, what happens to

Stroke volume?

Increases

Vessel compliance?

Decreases

Heart rate?

Decreases

What enzyme is needed to activate the following reactions?

Trypsinogen to trypsin

Enterokinase

Chymotrypsinogen to chymotrypsin

Trypsin

Procarboxypeptidase to carboxypeptidase

Trypsin

In a ventricular pacemaker cell, what phase of the action potential is affected by ACh?

Phase 4; ACh hyperpolarizes the cell via increasing potassium conductance, taking longer to reach threshold and slowing the rate of firing.

What is the most potent stimulus for glucagon secretion? Inhibition?

Hypoglycemia for **secretion** and **hyper**glycemia for **inhibition**

What is the term for the summation of mechanical stimuli due to the skeletal muscle contractile unit becoming saturated with calcium?

Tetany

What form of renal tubular reabsorption is characterized by low back leaks, high affinity of a substance, and easy saturation? It is surmised that the entire filtered load is reabsorbed until the carriers are saturated, and then the rest is excreted.

A transport maximum (Tm) system

In an *adrenergic nerve* terminal, where is dopamine converted to NE? By what enzyme?

Dopamine is converted into NE in the **vesicle** via the *enzyme* **dopamine-β-hydroxylase.**

Is the clearance for a substance greater than or less than for inulin if it is freely filtered and secreted? If it is freely filtered and reabsorbed?

Filtered and secreted: $C_x > C_{in}$ (i.e., PAH). Filtered and reabsorbed: $C_x < C_{in}$ (i.e., glucose), where C_x = clearance of a substance and C_{in} = clearance of inulin.

What is the term for the load on a muscle in the *relaxed state*?

Preload. It is the **load** on a muscle **P**rior to contraction.

The surge of what hormone induces ovulation?

LH

What are the two *best* indices of left ventricular preload?

LVEDV and LVEDP (left ventricular end-diastolic volume and end-diastolic pressure, respectively)

What stage of male development is characterized by the following LH and testosterone levels?

LH pulsatile amplitude and levels increase, with increased testosterone production.	Puberty
Both LH and testosterone levels drop and remain low.	Childhood
LH secretion drives testosterone production, with both levels paralleling each other.	Adulthood
Decreased testosterone production is accompanied by an increase in LH production.	Aged adult

Why is the clearance of creatinine always slightly greater than the clearance of inulin and GFR?

Because creatinine is filtered and a small amount is secreted

What primary acid-base disturbance is caused by a *loss in fixed acid* forcing the reaction to *shift to the right,* thereby *increasing* HCO_3^- levels?

Metabolic **alk**alosis (summary: **high pH, low H^+ and high HCO_3^-**)

When referring to a series circuit, what happens to resistance when a *resistor* is *added*?

Resistance **increases** as resistors are added to the circuit.

Why is there an increase in prolactin if the hypothalamic-pituitary axis was severed?

Because the chronic *inhibition* of **dopamine** (PIF) on the release of prolactin from the anterior pituitary gland is *removed,* thereby *increasing* the secretion of **prolactin**.

What acid form of H^+ in the urine cannot be titrated?

NH^{4+} (ammonium)

Regarding the venous system, what happens to blood volume if there is a small change in pressure?

Because the venous system is more **compliant** than the arterial vessels, small changes in pressure result in **large changes in blood volume.**

In what stage of sleep is GH secreted?

Stages 3 and 4 (NREM)

Where does the conversion of CO_2 into HCO_3^- take place?

In the RBC; remember, you need carbonic anhydrase for the conversion, and plasma does not have this enzyme.

From the fourth month of fetal life to term, what secretes the progesterone and estrogen to maintains the uterus?

The placenta

What two factors are required for effective exocytosis?

Calcium and **ATP** are required for packaged macromolecules to be extruded from the cell.

What is the best measure of total body vitamin D if you suspect a deficiency?

Serum 25-hydroxy-vitamin D (25-OH-D)

What hormone is required for 1,25-dihydroxy-vitamin D (1,25-diOH-D) to have bone resorbing effects?

PTH

Is bone deposition or resorption due to increased interstitial Ca^{2+} concentrations?

Bone **deposition** increases with **increased** Ca^{2+} or PO_4^- concentrations, whereas **resorption** (breakdown) is increased when there are **low levels** of Ca^{2+} or PO_4^-.

The opening of what valve indicates the termination of *isovolumetric relaxation* phase of the cardiac cycle?

Opening of the **mitral valve** indicates the termination of the isovolumetric relaxation phase and the beginning of the ventricular filling phase.

Why is there a decrease in the production in epinephrine when the anterior pituitary gland is removed?

The enzyme phenyl ethanolamine *N*-methyltransferase (PNMT), used in the conversion of epinephrine, is regulated by cortisol. Removing the anterior pituitary gland decreases ACTH and therefore cortisol.

Name the period described by the following statement: no matter how strong a stimulus is, no further action potentials can be stimulated.

Absolute refractory period is due to voltage inactivation of sodium channels.

How many carbons do estrogens have?

Estrogens are 18-carbon steroids. (Removal of one carbon from an androgen produces an estrogen.)

True or false? The alveolar P_{O_2} and P_{CO_2} levels match the pulmonary end capillary blood levels.

True. Because of intrapulmonary shunting, there is a slight decrease in P_{O_2} and increase in P_{CO_2} between the pulmonary end capillary blood and the systemic arterial blood.

In high altitudes, what is the main drive for ventilation?

The main drive shifts from central chemoreceptors (CSF H^+) to **peripheral chemoreceptors monitoring low P_{O_2}** levels.

Describe what type of fluid is either gained or lost with the following changes in body hydration for the ECF volume, ICF volume, and body osmolarity, respectively:

ECF, decrease; ICF, no change; body, no change

Loss of **isotonic** fluid (diarrhea, vomiting, hemorrhage)

ECF, increase; ICF, increase; body, decrease	**Gain of hypotonic** fluid (water intoxication or hypotonic saline)
ECF, decrease; ICF, decrease; body: increase	**Loss of hypotonic** fluid (alcohol, diabetes insipidus, dehydration)
ECF: increase; ICF: no change; body: no change	**Gain of isotonic** fluid (isotonic saline)
ECF, increase; ICF, decrease; body, increase	**Gain of hypertonic** fluid (mannitol or hypertonic saline)

What hormone excess produces adrenal hyperplasia?

ACTH

Is there more circulating T_3 or T_4 in plasma?

T_4; because of the greater affinity for the binding protein, T_4 has a significantly (nearly fifty times) longer half-life than T_3.

Why is the cell's resting membrane potential negative?

The resting membrane potential of the cell is **−90 mV** because of the intracellular **proteins.**

True or false? Thyroid size is a measure of its function.

False. Thyroid size is a measure of TSH levels (which are goitrogenic).

If the radius of a vessel is *decreased* by half, what happens to the resistance?

The resistance **increases** 16-fold.

What neurotransmitter is essential for maintaining a normal BP when an individual is standing?

NE, via its vasoconstrictive action on blood vessels

What form of diabetes insipidus is due to an *insufficient amount* of ADH for the renal collecting ducts?

Central/neurogenic diabetes insipidus; in the nephrogenic form there is sufficient ADH available, but the renal collecting ducts are impermeable to its actions.

Name the three methods of *vasodilation* via the

1. Decrease α-1 activity
2. Increase β-2 activity

sympathetic nervous system.

3. Increase ACh levels

What hormone is characterized by the following renal effects?

Calcium reabsorption, phosphate excretion

PTH

Calcium excretion, phosphate excretion

Calcitriol

Calcium reabsorption, phosphate reabsorption

Vitamin D_3

True or false? Progesterone has thermogenic activities.

True. Elevated plasma levels of progesterone can raise the body temperature 0.5° to 1.0°F.

How long is the transit time through the small intestine?

2 to 4 hours

Where is the last conducting zone of the lungs?

Terminal bronchioles. (No gas exchange occurs here.)

True or false? Cortisol inhibits glucose uptake in skeletal muscle.

True; cortisol inhibits glucose uptake in most tissue, making it available for neural tissue use.

What percentage of cardiac output flows through the pulmonary circuit?

100%; the percentage of blood flow through the pulmonary and systemic circulations are equal.

Name the Hgb-O_2 binding site based on the following information:

Least affinity for O_2; requires the highest PO_2 levels for attachment (approx. 100 mm Hg)

Site 4

Greatest affinity of the three remaining sites for attachment; requires Po$_2$ levels of 26 mm Hg to remain attached	Site 2
Remains attached under most physiologic conditions	Site 1
Requires a Po$_2$ level of 40 mm Hg to remain attached	Site 3
Which three factors cause the release of epinephrine from the adrenal medulla?	1. Exercise 2. Emergencies (stress) 3. Exposure to cold (The three **E**s)
How many ATPs are hydrolyzed every time a skeletal muscle cross-bridge completes a single cycle?	One, and it provides the **energy** for **mechanical contraction**.
Why would a puncture to a vein *above the heart* have the potential to introduce air into the vascular system?	Venous pressure *above the heart is **subatmospheric**,* so a puncture there has the potential to introduce air into the system.
What type of saliva is produced under parasympathetic stimulation?	High volume, watery solution; sympathetic stimulation results in thick, mucoid saliva.
In what area of the GI tract does iron get absorbed?	Duodenum
Why is the apex of the lung hypoventilated when a person is standing upright?	The alveoli at the apex are **almost completely inflated prior to inflation**, and although they are large, they receive **low levels of alveolar ventilation**.

What pancreatic islet cell secretes glucagons?

α-Cells; glucagon has *stimulatory effects* on β-cells and *inhibitory effects* on δ-cells.

What are the four characteristics of all *protein-mediated transportation*?

1. **Competition for carrier** with similar chemical substances
2. **Chemical specificity** needed for transportation
3. **Zero-order saturation kinetics** (Transportation is maximal when all transporters are saturated.)
4. Rate of **transportation faster** than if by simple diffusion

What is secretin's pancreatic action?

Secretin stimulates the pancreas to secrete a **HCO_3^--rich solution** to neutralize the acidity of the chyme entering the duodenum.

Why is there an increase in FF if the GFR is decreased under sympathetic stimulation?

Because **RPF** is **markedly decreased,** while **GFR** is only **minimally diminished;** this results in an **increase in FF** (remember $FF = GFR/RPF$).

What triggers phase 3 of the action potential in a ventricular pacemaker cell?

Rapid efflux of potassium

What is the primary target for the action of glucagon?

Liver (hepatocytes)

What is the renal compensation mechanism for acidosis?

Production of HCO_3^-, **shifting the reaction to the left** and thereby **decreasing H^+**

What enzyme found in a *cholinergic synapse* breaks down *ACh*? What are the byproducts?

Acetylcholinesterase breaks **ACh** into **acetate** and **choline** (which gets *resorbed* by the presynaptic nerve terminal).

What hormone, produced by Sertoli cells, if absent would result in the formation of internal female structures?

MIF

What happens to the lung if the intrapleural pressure exceeds lung recoil?

The lung will expand; also the opposite is true.

What two factors determine the clearance of a substance?

Plasma concentration and excretion rate

What type of muscle contraction occurs when the muscle shortens and lifts the load placed on it?

Isotonic contraction

What type of potential is characterized as being an all-or-none response, propagated and not summated?

Action potential

What primary acid-base disturbance is caused by a *gain in fixed acid* forcing the reaction to *shift to the left*, decreasing HCO_3^- and slightly *increasing CO_2*?

Metabolic **acid**osis (summary: **low pH, high H^+, and low HCO_3^-**)

What two pituitary hormones are produced by acidophils?

GH and **prolactin** are produced by **acidophils;** all others are by basophils.

What organ of the body has the smallest AV oxygen difference?

The **renal circulation** has the smallest AV O_2 (high venous PO_2) difference in the body because of the overperfusion of the kidneys resulting from filtration.

What is the titratable acid form of H^+ in the urine?

$H_2PO_4^-$ (dihydrogen phosphate)

What hypothalamic hormone is synthesized in the *preoptic nucleus*?

GnRH

What five factors promote turbulent flow?

1. Increased tube radius
2. Increased velocity

3. Decreased viscosity
4. Increased number of branches
5. Narrowing of an orifice

What is the major hormone produced in the following areas of the adrenal cortex?

Zona glomerulosa   Aldosterone

Zona fasciculata   Cortisol

Zona reticularis   DHEA (androgens)
Remember, from the outer cortex to the inner layer, **Salt, Sugar, Sex**. The adrenal cortex gets sweeter as you go deeper.

Where is most of the body's Ca^{2+} stored?   In bone; nearly 99% of Ca^{2+} is stored in the bone as hydroxyapatite.

What is the relationship between ventilation and Pco_2 levels?   They are inversely related. If **ventilation increases,** there will be a **decrease in Pco_2** levels and vice versa.

Is T_3 or T_4 responsible for the negative feedback loop on to the hypothalamus and anterior pituitary gland? T_4, as long as T_4 levels remain constant, TSH will be minimally effected by T_3.

What is the signal to open the voltage-gated transmembrane *potassium* channels?   **Membrane depolarization** is the stimulus to open these slow channels, and if they are prevented from opening, it will slow down the repolarization phase.

Increased urinary excretion of what substance is used to detect excess bone demineralization?   Hydroxyproline

What is the term to describe how easily a vessel stretches?   Compliance (think of it as distensibility)

What is the ratio of T_4:T_3 secretion from the thyroid gland?

20:1T_4T_3. There is an increase in the production of T_3 when iodine becomes deficient.

Do the PO_2 peripheral chemoreceptors of the carotid body contribute to the *normal drive* for ventilation?

Under normal resting conditions **no,** but they are *strongly stimulated* when PO_2 arterial levels **decrease to 50 to 60 mm Hg,** resulting in increased ventilatory drive.

What determines the overall force generated by the ventricular muscle during systole?

The number of cross-bridges cycling during contraction: the **greater** the number, the **greater** the force of contraction.

Where does most circulating plasma epinephrine originate?

From the adrenal medulla; NE is mainly derived from the postsynaptic sympathetic neurons.

What causes a skeletal muscle contraction to terminate?

When **calcium** is removed from troponin and *pumped* back into the **SR,** skeletal muscle contraction stops.

What happens to intracellular volume when there is an *increase* in osmolarity?

ICF volume **decreases** when there is an **increase** in osmolarity and vice versa.

Which CHO is independently absorbed from the small intestine?

Fructose; both glucose and galactose are actively absorbed via secondary active transport.

When is the surface tension the greatest in the respiratory cycle?

Surface tension, the force to collapse the lung, is greatest **at the end of inspiration.**

What adrenal enzyme deficiency results in hypertension, hypernatremia, increased ECF volume, and decreased adrenal androgen production?

17-α-Hydroxylase deficiency

In reference to membrane potential (Em) and equilibrium potential (Ex), which way do ions diffuse?	Ions diffuse in the direction to bring the membrane potential toward the equilibrium potential.
Under normal conditions, what is the main factor that determines GFR?	Hydrostatic pressure of the glomerular capillaries (promotes filtration)
The closure of what valve indicates the beginning of the *isovolumetric relaxation* phase of the cardiac cycle?	Closure of the **aortic valve** indicates the termination of the ejection phase and the beginning of the isovolumetric relaxation phase of the cardiac cycle.
What vessels in the systemic circulation have the greatest and slowest velocity?	The **aorta** has the **greatest** velocity and the **capillaries** have the **slowest** velocity.
Thin extremities, fat collection on the upper back and abdomen, hypertension, hypokalemic alkalosis, acne, hirsutism, wide purple striae, osteoporosis, hyperlipidemia, hyperglycemia with insulin resistance, and protein depletion are all characteristics of what disorder?	Hypercortisolism (Cushing syndrome)
What enzyme is essential for the conversion of CO_2 to HCO_3^-?	Carbonic anhydrase
True or false? The parasympathetic nervous system has very little effect on arteriolar dilation or constriction.	True

What three lung measurements must be calculated because they cannot be measured by simple spirometry?

TLC, FRC, and RV have to be calculated. (Remember, any volume that has RV as a component has be calculated.)

What is the venous and arterial stretch receptors' function regarding the secretion of ADH?

They **chronically inhibit** ADH secretion; when there is a **decrease** in the blood volume, the stretch receptors send **fewer signals,** and ADH is secreted.

What cell converts androgens to estrogens?

Granulosa cell

What hormone acts on this cell?

FSH

How long is the transit time through the large intestine?

3 to 4 days

Does subatmospheric pressure act to expand or collapse the lung?

Subatmospheric pressure acts to **expand** the lung; **positive pressure** acts to **collapse** the lung.

What hormone constricts afferent and efferent arterioles (efferent more so) in an effort to preserve glomerular capillary pressure as the renal blood flow decreases?

AT II

Why is there a minimal change in BP during exercise if there is a large drop in TPR?

Because the **large drop in TPR** is accompanied by a **large increase in cardiac output,** resulting in a minimal change in BP.

What is the effect of insulin on protein storage?

Insulin **increases** total body stores of protein, fat, and CHOs. When you think insulin, you think **storage.**

What is the term for an inhibitory interneuron?

Renshaw neuron

What triggers phase 0 of the action potential in a ventricular pacemaker cell?

Calcium influx secondary to slow channel opening

What are the following changes seen in the luminal fluid by the time it leaves the PCT of the nephron?

Percentage of original filtered volume left in the lumen

At the end of the PCT 25% of the original volume is left

Percentage of Na^+, Cl^-, K^+ left in the lumen

At the end of the PCT 25% of Na^+, Cl^-, K^+ is left

Osmolarity

300 mOsm/L

Concentration of CHO, AA, ketones, peptides

No CHO, AA, ketones, or peptides are left in the tubular lumen.

True or false? Enterokinase is a brush border enzyme.

False. It is an enzyme secreted by the lining of the small intestine.

Where does the synthesis of ACh occur?

In the **cytoplasm** of the presynaptic nerve terminal; it is *catalyzed* by **choline acetyltransferase.**

What pancreatic islet cell secretes *somatostatin*?

δ-Cells; somatostatin has an *inhibitory effect* on **α-** and **β-islet cells.**

Why is O_2 *content* depressed in anemic patients?

Anemic patients have a **depressed O_2 content** because of the **reduced concentration of Hgb** in the blood. As for **polycythemic** patients, their **O_2 content is increased** because of the **excess Hgb concentrations.**

What term describes the volume of plasma from which a substance is removed over time?

Clearance

If capillary *hydrostatic pressure* is *greater than oncotic pressure*, is filtration or reabsorption promoted?

Filtration; if hydrostatic pressure is **less than** oncotic pressure, **reabsorption** is promoted.

What cells of the parathyroid gland are simulated in response to *hypo*calcemia?

The **chief cells** of the parathyroid gland release **PTH** in response to **hypocalcemia**.

At the base of the lung, what is the baseline intrapleural pressure, and what force does it exert on the alveoli?

Intrapleural pressure at the base is **−2.5 cm H₂O (more positive** than the mean), resulting in a force to **collapse the alveoli.**

What hormone is necessary for normal GH secretion?

Normal thyroid hormones levels in the plasma are necessary for proper secretion of GH. Hypothyroid patients have decreased GH secretions.

What is the signal to open the voltage-gated transmembrane *sodium* channels?

Membrane depolarization is the stimulus to open these channels, which are closed in resting conditions.

What hormones are *produced* in the *median eminence* region of the hypothalamus and the *posterior pituitary* gland?

None; they are the *storage* sites for ADH and oxytocin.

What is the most energy-demanding phase of the cardiac cycle?

Isovolumetric contraction

What presynaptic receptor does NE use to terminate further neurotransmitter release?

α_2-Receptors

Are salivary secretions hypertonic, hypotonic, or isotonic?

Hypotonic, because NaCl is reabsorbed in the salivary ducts

What is the effect of T_3 on *heart rate* and *cardiac output*?

T_3 **increases** both heart rate and cardiac output by **increasing** the number of **β-receptors** and their **sensitivity** to catecholamines.

Why will turbulence first appear in the aorta in patients with anemia?

Because it is the **largest vessel** and has the **highest velocity** in systemic circulation

What is the origin of the polyuria if a patient is dehydrated and electrolyte depleted?

If the polyuria begins **before the collecting ducts,** the patient is dehydrated and **electrolyte depleted**. If the polyuria originates **from the collecting ducts,** the patient is dehydrated with **normal electrolytes.**

What is the physiologically active form of Ca^{2+}?

Free ionized Ca^{2+}

What are the two factors that affect alveolar P_{CO_2} levels?

Metabolic rate and alveolar ventilation (main factor)

Why is spermatogenesis decreased with anabolic steroid therapy?

Exogenous steroids suppress LH release and result in Leydig cell atrophy. Testosterone, produced by Leydig cells, is needed for spermatogenesis.

What type of membrane is characterized as being permeable to *water only*?

Semipermeable membrane; a selectively permeable membrane allows both water and small solutes to pass through its membrane.

What thyroid enzyme is needed for *oxidation* of $I-$ to I'?

Peroxidase, which is also needed for **iodination** and **coupling** inside the follicular cell

What is the most important stimulus for the secretion of insulin?

An increase in serum glucose levels

What term is described as the prestretch on the ventricular muscle at the end of diastole?

Preload (the load on the muscle in the relaxed state)

What peripheral chemoreceptor receives the most blood per gram of weight in the body?

The carotid body, which monitors arterial blood directly

What adrenal enzyme deficiency results in hypertension, hypernatremia, and virilization?

11-β-Hydroxylase deficiency results in **excess** production of **11-deoxycorticosterone,** a weak mineralocorticoid. It increases BP, Na^+, and ECF volume along with production of adrenal androgens.

What is the term for diffusion of water across a semipermeable or selectively permeable membrane?

Osmosis; water will diffuse from **higher** to **lower water** concentrations.

When do hCG concentrations peak in pregnancy?

In the first 3 months

How many milliliters of O_2 per milliliter of blood?

0.2

What type of cell is surrounded by mineralized bone?

Osteocyte

What two forces affect movement of ions across a membrane?

Concentration force and electrical force

What happens to the resistance of the system when a resistor is added in a series?

Resistance of the system **increases.** (Remember, when resistors are **connected in a series,** the total of the **resistance** is the **sum of the individual resistances.**)

What is the greatest component of lung recoil?

Surface tension; in the alveoli, it is a force that acts to collapse the lung.

Where is ADH synthesized?

In the supraoptic nuclei of the hypothalamus; it is stored in the posterior pituitary gland.

How is velocity related to the total cross-sectional area of a blood vessel?

Velocity is **inversely related** to cross-sectional area.

True or false? Aldosterone has a sodium-conserving action in the distal colon.

True. In the distal colon, sweat glands, and salivary ducts, aldosterone has sodium-conserving effects.

What form of hormone is described as having membrane-bound receptors that are stored in vesicles, using second messengers, and having its activity determined by free hormone levels.

Water-soluble hormones are considered **fast-acting hormones.**

What forms of fatty acids are absorbed from the small intestine mucosa by *simple diffusion*?

Short-chain fatty acids

What is the term for the day after the LH surge in the female cycle?

Ovulation

The opening of what valve indicates the beginning of the *ejection phase* of the cardiac cycle?

Opening of the **aortic valve** terminates the isovolumetric phase and begins the ejection phase of the cardiac cycle.

What is the region of an axon where no myelin is found?

Nodes of Ranvier

What disorder of aldosterone secretion is characterized by

    ***Increased* total body sodium, ECF volume, plasma volume, BP, and pH; *decreased* potassium, renin and AT II activity; *no edema*?**

Primary hyperaldosteronism (Conn syndrome)

Decreased total body sodium, ECF volume, plasma volume, BP, and pH; *increased* potassium, renin, and AT II activity; *no edema?*	Primary hypoaldosteronism (Addison's disease)

What four factors affect diffusion rate?

1. Concentration (**greater** concentration gradient, **greater** diffusion rate)
2. Surface area (**greater** surface area, **greater** diffusion rate)
3. Solubility (**greater** solubility, **greater** diffusion rate)
4. Membrane thickness (**thicker** the membrane, **slower** the diffusion rate)

Molecular weight is clinically **unimportant.**

How long after ovulation does fertilization occur?

8 to 25 hours

What is the name of the force that develops in the wall of the lungs as they expand?

Lung recoil, being a force to collapse the lung, **increases as the lung enlarges** during inspiration.

What day of the menstrual cycle does ovulation take place?

Day 14

How does sympathetic stimulation to the skin result in decreased blood flow and decreased blood volume? (Hint: what vessels are stimulated, and how?)

A decrease in cutaneous **blood flow** results from **constriction of the arterioles,** and decreased cutaneous **blood volume** results from **constriction of the venous plexus**.

What two compensatory mechanisms occur to reverse hypoxia at high altitudes?

Increase in erythropoietin and increase in 2,3-BPG, also called 2,3-diphosphoglycerate (2,3-P$_2$Gri) (increase in glycolysis)

What female follicular cell is under LH stimulation and produces androgens from cholesterol?

Theca cell

What is the main factor determining FF?

Renal plasma flow (**decrease** flow, **increase** FF)

Where is the action potential generated on a neuron?

Axon hillock

If free water clearance (CH_2O) is positive, what type of urine is formed? And if is negative?

If *positive,* hypotonic urine (osmolarity < 300 mOsm/L); if *negative,* hypertonic urine (osmolarity > 300 mOsm/L)>>

What cell in the heart has the highest rate of automaticity?

SA node; it is the reason it is the primary pacemaker of the heart.

What is pumped from the lumen of the ascending loop of Henle to decrease the osmolarity?

NaCl is removed from the lumen to dilute the fluid leaving the loop of Henle.

True or false? In skeletal muscle relaxation is an active event.

True. Sarcoplasmic calcium-dependent ATPase supplies the *energy* to **terminate contraction,** and therefore it is an **active** process.

What three factors increase simple diffusion?

1. Increased solubility
2. Increased concentration gradient
3. Decreased thickness of the membrane

What is the pancreatic action of CKK?

CCK stimulates the pancreas to release **amylase, lipase,** and **proteases** for digestion.

What is the *rate-limiting step* in a conduction of a NMJ?

The time it takes **ACh** to *diffuse* to the postjunctional membrane

Is excretion greater than or less than filtration for net secretion to occur?

Excretion is greater than filtration for net secretion to occur.

What acid-base disturbance is produced from *vomiting*?

Hypokalemic metabolic alkalosis occurs from vomiting because of the loss of H^+, K^+, and Cl^-.

What phase of the menstrual cycle is dominated by estrogen? Progesterone?

Follicular phase is **estrogen-**dependent with increased FSH levels, while the **luteal** phase is **progesterone-**dependent.

Name the lung measurement based on the following descriptions:

    The amount of air that enters or leaves the lung system in a single breath

Tidal volume (V_T)

    The maximal volume inspired from FRC

Inspiratory capacity

    Additional volume that can be expired after normal expiration

ERV

    Maximal volume that can be expired after maximal inspiration

VC

    Volume in the lungs at the end of passive expiration

FRC

    Additional air that can be taken in after normal inspiration

IRV

    Amount of air in the lungs after maximal expiration

RV

Amount of air in the lungs after maximal inspiration	TLC
What growth factors are chondrogenic, working on the epiphyseal end plates of bone?	Somatomedins (IGF-1)
What determines the V_{max} of skeletal muscle?	The muscle's ATPase activity
True or false? All of the hormones in the hypothalamus and anterior pituitary gland are water soluble.	True
What is the effect of T_3 on the glucose absorption in the small intestine?	Thyroid hormones **increase** serum glucose levels by increasing the absorption of glucose from the small intestine.
Is the bound form or free form of a lipid-soluble hormone responsible for the negative feedback activity?	**Free form** determines hormone activity and is responsible for the negative feedback loop.
What region or regions of the adrenal cortex are stimulated by ACTH?	Zona fasciculata and zona reticularis
Are the following parameters associated with an obstructive or restrictive lung disorder: *decreased* FEV_1, FVC, peak flow, and FEV_1/FVC; *increased* TLC, FRC, and RV?	**Obstructive** lung disorders. The opposite changes (where you see decrease exchange it for increase and vice versa) are seen in a **restrictive** pattern.
What is the respiratory compensation mechanism for metabolic alkalosis?	**Hypo**ventilation, which **increases CO_2, shifting the reaction to the right** and **increasing H^+**

During puberty, what is the main drive for the increased GH secretion?

Increased androgen secretion at puberty drives the increased GH secretion.

What type of potential is characterized as graded, decremental, and exhibiting summation?

Subthreshold potential

What three organs are responsible for peripheral conversion of T_4 to T_3?

Liver, kidneys, and pituitary gland via 5' deiodinase enzyme

The closure of what valve indicates the beginning of *isovolumetric contraction*?

Mitral valve closure indicates the termination of the ventricular filling phase and beginning of isovolumetric contraction.

How many carbons do androgens have?

Androgens are 19-carbon steroids.

At the *apex* of the lung, what is the baseline intrapleural pressure, and what force does it exert on the alveoli?

Baseline apical intrapleural pressure is -10 cm H_2O (**more negative** than the mean) resulting in a force to **expand the alveoli.**

True or false? Renin secretion is *increased* in 21-β-hydroxylase deficiency.

True. Increased **renin** and **AT II** levels occur as a result of the **decreased** production of **aldosterone**.

What are the four ways to *increase* TPR?

1. Decrease the radius of the vessel
2. Increase the length of the vessel
3. Increase the viscosity
4. Decrease the number of parallel channels

What form of estrogen is of placental origin?

Estriol

What term is an index of the effort needed to expand the lungs (i.e., overcomes recoil)?

Compliance; the more compliant a lung is, the easier it is to inflate.

At which three sites in the body is T$_4$ converted to T$_3$?

1. Liver
2. Kidney
3. Pituitary gland (via 5'-deiodinase enzyme)

Using Laplace's relationship regarding wall tension, why is the wall tension in an aneurysm greater than in the surrounding normal blood vessel's wall?

The wall tension is **greater** because the aneurysm has a **greater** radius than the surrounding vessel.

What percentage of nephrons is cortical?

Seven-eighths of nephrons are cortical, with the remainder juxtamedullary.

To what is the diffusion rate indirectly proportional?

Diffusion rate is **indirectly** proportional to **membrane thickness** and is **directly** proportional to **membranes surface area.**

ADH is secreted in response to what two stimuli?

ADH is secreted in response to *increased* **plasma osmolarity** and *decreased* **blood volume**.

What vessels have the *largest total* cross-sectional area in systemic circulation?

Capillaries

How many days before the first day of menstrual bleeding is ovulation?

14 days in most women (Remember, the luteal phase is always constant.)

What is the major muscle used in the relaxed state of expiration?

Under resting conditions expiration is considered a **passive process;** therefore, **no muscles** are used. In the **active state** the **abdominal muscles** can be considered the major muscle of expiration.

What subunit of hCG is used to detect whether a patient is pregnant?

The β-subunit; remember, the α-subunit is nonspecific.

What happens to capillary oncotic pressure with dehydration?

Oncotic pressure **increases** because of the removal of water.

What cells of the kidney are extravascular chemoreceptors for decreased Na^+, Cl^-, and NaCl?

Macula densa

What is the effect of insulin on intracellular K^+ stores?

Insulin **increases intracellular** K^+ stores while **decreasing serum** K^+ levels.

What triggers phase 4 of the action potential in a ventricular pacemaker cell?

Decreasing potassium conductance, which results in increased excitability

What is it called when levels of sex steroids increase, LH increases, and FSH increases?

GnRH pulsatile infusion

What parasympathetic neurotransmitter of the GI tract stimulates the release of *gastrin*?

Gastrin-releasing peptide (GRP) stimulates **G** cells to release **g**astrin. (All **G**'s)

What reflex increases TPR in an attempt to maintain BP during a hemorrhage?

The carotid sinus reflex

What is the name of the regulatory protein that covers the attachment site on actin in resting skeletal muscle?

Tropomyosin

Which way does the Hgb-O_2 dissociation curve shift in patients with CO poisoning?

The pathologic problem with CO poisoning is that CO has **240 times as much affinity for Hgb** molecule as does O_2, **reducing the carrying capacity** and **shifting the curve to the left,** making it difficult to remove the CO molecule from Hgb.

What is the main factor determining GFR?

Glomerular capillary pressure (**increased** glomerular capillary pressure, **increased GFR and vice versa**)

What is the effect of hypoventilation on cerebral blood flow?

Hypoventilation results in an **increase in Pco_2 levels** and therefore an **increase in blood flow.**

What cells of the thyroid gland are stimulated in response to *hyper*calcemia?

The **parafollicular cells** of the thyroid (C cells) release **calcitonin** in response to **hypercalcemia.**

What is the term for the amount of blood in the ventricle after *maximal* contraction?

Residual volume

What does failure of Pao_2 to increase with supplemental O_2 indicate?

Pulmonary shunt (i.e., pulmonary embolism)

What two substances stimulate Sertoli cells?

FSH and testosterone

The clearance of what substance is the *gold standard* of RPF?

PAH

What bile pigment is formed by the metabolism of bilirubin by intestinal bacteria, giving stool its brown color?

Stercobilin

Is ACh associated with bronchoconstriction or bronchodilation?

Bronchoconstriction is associated with **parasympathetic** stimulation (ACh), and **catecholamine** stimulation is associated with **bronchodilation** (why epinephrine is used in emergency treatment of bronchial asthma.)

What are the growth factors released from the liver called?

Somatomedins

Regarding skeletal muscle mechanics, what is the relationship between velocity and afterload?

An increase in the afterload decreases velocity; they are inversely related. (V equals 1 divided by afterload.)

What happens to extracellular volume with a net *gain* in body fluid?

The ECF compartment always **enlarges** when there is a **net gain** in total body water and decreases when there is a loss of total body water. Hydration status is named in terms of the ECF compartment.

What are the six substances that promote the secretion of insulin?

1. Glucose
2. Amino acid (arginine)
3. Gastrin inhibitory peptide (GIP)
4. Glucagon
5. β-Agonists
6. ACh

Does O_2 or CO_2 have a *higher driving force* across the alveolar membrane?

O_2 has a higher driving force but is only one-twenty-fourth as soluble as CO_2. CO_2 has a very small partial pressure difference across the alveolar membrane $(47 - 40 = 7 \text{ mmHg})$, but it is extremely soluble and therefore diffuses readily across the membrane.

What is used as an index for both adrenal and testicular androgens?

Urinary 17-ketosteroids

How are resistance and length related regarding flow?

Resistance and vessel length are **proportionally** related. The **greater** the **length** of the vessel, the **greater** the **resistance** is on the vessel.

Is filtration greater than or less than excretion for net reabsorption to occur?

Filtration is greater than excretion for net reabsorption to occur.

What hormone, stimulated by epinephrine, results in an increase in lipolysis?

Hormone-sensitive lipase, which breaks down triglyceride into glycerol and free fatty acid

True or false? Miniature end-plate potentials (MEPPs) generate action potentials.

False

Is GH considered a gluconeogenic hormone?

Yes, it *decreases* **fat and muscle** *uptake* of glucose, thereby increasing blood glucose levels.

True or false? Somatic motor neurons innervate the striated muscle of the bulbospongiosus and ischiocavernous muscles and result in ejaculation of semen.

True

What happens to intraventricular pressure and volume during isovolumetric contraction?

As the name indicates, there is **no change in volume** but there is an **increase in pressure**.

Do high levels of estrogen and progesterone block milk synthesis?

Yes, they stimulate the growth of mammary tissue but block milk synthesis. At parturition, the decrease in estrogen lifts the block on milk production.

What two factors lead to the development of the bends (caisson disease)?

Breathing high-pressure nitrogen over a long time and sudden decompression result in the bends.

In what type of circuit is the total resistance *always less* than that of the individual resistors?

Parallel circuit

What is the term for days 15 to 28 in the female cycle?

Luteal phase

What happens to total and alveolar ventilation with

Increased rate of breathing?

With an increased rate of breathing the total ventilation is greater than the alveolar ventilation. Rapid, shallow breathing increases dead space ventilation with little change in alveolar ventilation. (This is *hypo*ventilation).

Increased depth of breathing?

With an increased depth of breathing both the total and alveolar ventilation increase.
This concept is always tested on the boards, so *remember it*.

What pathophysiologic disorder is characterized by the following changes in cortisol and ACTH?

Cortisol decreased, ACTH increased

Primary **hypo**cortisolism (Addison's disease)

Cortisol increased, ACTH increased

Secondary **hyper**cortisolism (pituitary)

Cortisol increased, ACTH decreased

Primary **hyper**cortisolism

Cortisol decreased, ACTH decreased

Secondary **hypo**cortisolism (pituitary)

What happens to flow and pressure in capillaries with arteriolar dilation? Arteriolar constriction?

Capillary flow and pressure **increase** with arteriolar dilation and **decrease** with arteriolar constriction.

What has occurred to the renal arterioles based on the following changes in the GFR, RPF, FF, and glomerular capillary pressure?

GFR ↑, RPF ↑, FF normal, capillary pressure ↑	Dilation of afferent arteriole
GFR ↑, RPF ↓, FF ↑, capillary pressure ↑	Constriction of efferent arteriole
GFR ↓, RPF ↑, FF ↓, capillary pressure ↓	Dilation of efferent arteriole
GFR ↓, RPF ↓, FF normal, capillary pressure ↓	Constriction of afferent arteriole

Which direction is air flowing when the intra-alveolar pressure is zero?

When the intra-alveolar pressure equals zero, there is **no airflow.**

What phase of the female cycle occurs during days 1 to 15?

Follicular phase

What determines the effective osmolarity of the ICF and the ECF compartments?

The **concentration of plasma proteins** determines effective osmolarity because capillary membranes are freely permeable to all substances except proteins.

What region of the brain houses the central chemoreceptors responsible for control of ventilation?

The surface of the medulla

What is the site of action of *cholera* toxin?

Cholera toxin irreversibly activates the **cAMP-dependent chloride pumps** of the small and large intestine, producing a large volume of chloride-rich diarrhea.

Name the phase of the *ventricular muscle action potential* based on the following information:

Slow channels open, allowing calcium influx; voltage-gated potassium channels closed; potassium efflux through ungated channels; plateau stage	Phase 2
Slight repolarization secondary to potassium and closure of the sodium channels	Phase 1
Fast channels open, then quickly close, and sodium influx results in depolarization	Phase 0
Slow channels close, voltage-gated potassium channels reopen with a large influx of potassium, and the cell quickly repolarizes	Phase 3

Where in the kidney are the long loops of Henle and the terminal regions of the collecting ducts?

In the medulla; all the other structures are cortical.

What is absorbed in the gallbladder to concentrate bile?

Water

What type of hormone is described as having intracellular receptors, being synthesized as needed, mostly bound to

Lipid-soluble hormones are considered **slow-acting hormones**.

proteins, and having its activity determined by free hormone levels?

What are the three stimuli that result in the renin-angiotensin-aldosterone secretion?

1. Low pressure in the afferent renal arteriole
2. Low sodium sensed by the macula densa
3. Increased β-1-sympathetic stimulation of the JG cells

Is there a shift in p50 values with anemia? Polycythemia?

The p50 value does not change in either anemia or polycythemia; the main change is the carrying capacity of the blood.

What hormone level peaks 1 day before the surge of LH and FSH in the female cycle?

Estradiol

True or false? Active protein transport requires a concentration gradient.

True; it requires both a **concentration gradient** and **ATP** to work.

Up to how many hours post ejaculation do sperm retain their ability to fertilize the ovum?

Up to 72 hours; the ovum losses its ability to be fertilized 8 to 25 hours after release.

What type of membrane channel opens in response to depolarization?

Voltage-gated channel

What are the five effects of insulin on fat metabolism?

1. Increased glucose uptake by fat cells
2. Increased triglyceride uptake by fat cells
3. Increased conversion of CHOs into fat
4. Decreased lipolysis in fat tissue
5. Decreased ketone body formation

True or false? In a skeletal muscle fiber, the *interior* of the T-tubule is *extracellular.*

True. They are **evaginations** of the surface membranes and therefore extracellular.

Under resting conditions, what is the main determinant of cerebral blood flow?

Arterial P_{CO_2} levels are **proportional** to cerebral blood flow.

On the venous pressure curve, what do the following waves represent?

  A wave?

  Atrial contraction

  C wave?

  Ventricular **c**ontraction

  V wave?

  Atrial filling (**v**enous filling) **A**trial, **C**ontraction, **V**enous

What cell type in the bone is responsible for bone deposition?

Osteoblast (Remember, blasts make, clasts take)

True or false? The blood stored in the systemic veins and the pulmonary circuit are considered part of the cardiac output.

False. **Cardiac output** refers to *circulating blood volume.* The blood in the systemic veins and the pulmonary circuits are *storage reserves* and therefore are **not considered** in cardiac output.

What hormone disorder is characterized by the following abnormalities in sex steroids, LH, and FSH?

  Sex steroids ↓ , LH ↓ , FSH ↓

  Pituitary hypogonadism

  Sex steroids ↓ , LH ↓ , FSH ↓ ?

  GnRH constant infusion

  Sex steroids ↓ , LH ↑ , FSH ↑ ?

  Primary hypogonadism (postmenopausal women)

What are the three characteristics of autoregulation?

1. Flow independent of BP
2. Flow proportional to local metabolism
3. Flow independent of nervous reflexes

What is the fastest-conducting fiber of the heart? Slowest conduction fiber in the heart?	Purkinje cell is the fastest, and the AV node is the slowest.
What equals the total tension on a muscle minus the preload?	Afterload
What follicular cell possesses FSH receptors and converts androgens into estradiol?	Granulosa cells

What are the primary neurotransmitters at the following sites?

Postganglionic sympathetic neurons	NE
Chromaffin cells of the adrenal medulla	Epinephrine
Brainstem cells	Serotonin
The hypothalamus	Histamine
All motor neurons, postganglionic parasympathetic neurons	ACh
Autonomic preganglionic neurons	ACh
What region of the nephron has the highest osmolarity?	Tip of the loop of Henle (1200 mOsm/L)
What pH (acidotic or alkalotic) is needed for pepsinogen to pepsin conversion?	Acid is needed for the activation of pepsin and therefore needed for protein digestion.

What is the term for the amount of blood expelled from the ventricle per beat?

Stroke volume

True or false? Oxytocin *initiates* rhythmic contractions associated with labor.

False. It does *increase* uterine synthesis of **prostaglandins,** which increase uterine contractions.

Why does DLCO decrease in emphysema and fibrosis but increase during exercise?

DLCO, an index of lung surface area and membrane thickness, is **decreased in fibrosis** because of **increased membrane thickness** and **decreased in emphysema** because of increased surface area **without increase in capillary recruitment;** in **exercise** there is an **increase** in surface area due to **capillary recruitment.**

What enzyme converts androgens to estrogens?

Aromatase

The clearance of what substance is the *gold standard* of GFR?

Inulin

How does *myelination* affect conduction velocity of an action potential?

The **greater** the myelination, the **greater** the conduction velocity.

What are the three end products of amylase digestion?

1. Maltose
2. Maltotetrose
3. α-Limit dextrans (α-1,6 binding)

Where is most of the airway resistance in the respiratory system?

In the first and second bronchi

What is the respiratory compensation mechanism for metabolic acidosis?

Hyperventilation, which **decreases CO_2,** shifting the reaction to the left and **decreasing H^+**

How are resistance and viscosity related regarding flow?	Viscosity and resistance are **proportionally** related. The **greater** the **viscosity,** the **greater** the **resistance** is on the vessel.
T_3 increases bone ossification through synergistic effect with what hormone?	GH

Name the *ventricular muscle membrane channel*:

Closed* at rest; depolarization causes channels to open *slowly	Voltage-gated calcium channel
Always *open*	Ungated potassium channel
***Closed* at rest; depolarization causes channels to open *quickly*; will not respond to a second stimulus until cell is repolarized.**	Voltage-gated sodium channel
***Open* at rest; *depolarization* is stimulus to *close*; begin to reopen during the plateau phase and during repolarization**	Voltage-gated potassium channels
What are the three glycogenic organs?	Liver, kidney, and GI epithelium
Is CO_2 a perfusion- or diffusion-limited gas? O_2?	Since CO_2 is 24 times as soluble as O_2, the rate at which CO_2 is brought to the membrane determines its rate of exchange, making it a **perfusion-limited** gas. For O_2, the more time it is in contact with the membrane, the more likely it will diffuse, making it **diffusion-limited.**

What is the term for the potential difference across a cell membrane?

Transmembrane potential (an absolute number)

What adrenal enzyme deficiency can be summed up as a *mineralocorticoid* deficiency, *glucocorticoid* deficiency, and an *excess of adrenal androgens*?

21-β-Hydroxylase deficiency leads to **hypotension, hyponatremia,** and **virilization**.

When the ECF osmolarity *increases*, what happens to cell size?

Increase in ECF osmolarity means a **decrease** in ICF osmolarity, so cells **shrink.**

When does cortisol secretion peak?

In early-morning sleep, usually between the sixth and eighth hours

What is the term for ventilation of unperfused alveoli?

Alveolar dead space

What is the *bioactive* form of thyroid hormone?

T_3

What acid-base disturbance occurs in *colonic diarrhea*?

Hypokalemic metabolic acidosis occurs in colonic diarrhea because of the net secretion of HCO_3^- and potassium into the colonic lumen.

What two AAs act as excitatory transmitters in the CNS, generating EPSPs?

Glutamine and aspartate

What are the three mechanisms of action for atrial natriuretic peptide's diuretic and natriuretic affects?

1. Dilation of the afferent arteriole
2. Constriction of the efferent arteriole
3. Inhibition of reabsorption of sodium and water in the collecting ducts

In a parallel circuit, what happens to resistance when a resistor is added in *parallel*?

Resistance **decreases** as resistors are added in parallel.

What component of the ANS is responsible for movement of semen from the epididymis to the ejaculatory ducts?

Sympathetic nervous system

What happens to O$_2$ affinity with a decrease in p50?

O$_2$ affinity increases with a **decrease** in the **p50,** making O$_2$ **more difficult to remove** from the Hgb molecule.

If the ratio of a substance's filtrate and plasma concentrations are equal, what is that substance's affect on the kidney?

If the ratio of the filtrate to plasma concentration of a substance is equal, the substance is **freely filtered by the kidney.**

What does a *loss of afferent activity* from the carotid sinus onto the medulla signal?

A **loss** of afferent activity indicates a **decrease in BP,** and an **increase** in afferent activity indicates an **increase in BP.**

What are the five F's associated with gallstones?

1. **F**at
2. **F**orty
3. **F**emale
4. **F**amilial
5. **F**ertile

True or false? Menstruation is an *active* process due to *increased* gonadal sex hormones?

False. It is a **passive** process due to **decreased** sex hormones.

What happens to the intrapleural pressure when the diaphragm relaxes?

Relaxation of the diaphragm **increases** the intrapleural pressure (becomes more positive).

What component of the renin-angiotensin-aldosterone axis increases sodium reabsorption in the proximal convoluted tubules and increases *thirst drive*?

AT II

What large-diameter vessel has the *smallest* cross-sectional area in systemic circulation?	The aorta
Excess bone demineralization and remodeling can be detected by checking urine levels of what substance?	Hydroxyproline (breakdown product of collagen)
What happens to the following during skeletal muscle contraction?	
A band	No change in length
I band	Shortens
H zone	Shortens
Sarcomere	Shortens
Actin and myosin lengths	No change in length
What are the three effects of insulin on protein metabolism?	1. Increased amino acid uptake by muscles 2. Decreased protein breakdown 3. Increased protein synthesis
What is the main mechanism for exchange of nutrients and gases across a capillary membrane?	**Simple diffusion;** it does not use protein-mediated transport
What event signifies the first day of the menstrual cycle?	Onset of bleeding

Name the muscle type based on the histological features:

Actin and myosin in sarcomeres; striated; uninuclear; gap junctions; troponin:calcium binding complex; T tubules and SR forming dyadic contacts; voltage-gated calcium channels

Cardiac muscle

Actin and myosin in sarcomeres; striated; multinuclear; lacks gap junctions; troponin:calcium binding; T tubules and SR forming triadic contacts; highest ATPase activity; no calcium channels

Skeletal muscle

Actin and myosin not in sarcomeres; nonstriated; uninuclear; gap junctions; calmodulin:calcium binding; lacks T tubules; voltage-gated calcium channels

Smooth muscle

Name the valve abnormality based on the following criteria:

Back-filling into the left atrium during systole; increased v-wave, preload, left atrial volume, and left ventricular filling

Mitral insufficiency

Systolic murmur, increased preload and afterload, decreased aortic pulse pressure and coronary blood flow	Aortic stenosis
Diastolic murmur, increased right ventricular pressure, left atrial pressure, and atrial to ventricular pressure gradient; decreased left ventricular filling pressure	Mitral stenosis
Diastolic murmur; increased preload, stroke volume, and aortic pulse pressure; decreased coronary blood flow; no incisura; and peripheral vasodilation	Aortic insufficiency
Circulating levels of what hormone cause the cervical mucus to be thin and watery, allowing sperm an easier entry into the uterus?	Estrogen
What hormone controls relaxation of the lower esophageal sphincter during swallowing?	**VIP** is an inhibitory parasympathetic neurotransmitter that results in relaxation of the lower esophageal sphincter.
What is the term for the difference between systolic and diastolic pressures?	Pulse pressure
What hormone, produced by the *Sertoli* cells, is responsible for keeping testosterone levels in the seminiferous tubules nearly 50 times that of the serum?	Androgen-binding protein

True or false? There are no central O$_2$ receptors.

True

What cell type of the bone has PTH receptors?

Osteoblasts, which in turn stimulate osteoclasts to break down bone, releasing Ca^{2+} into the interstitium. (Remember, blasts make, clasts take.)

What substance is secreted by parietal gland and required for life?

Intrinsic factor (IF)

What is the only way to increase O$_2$ delivery in the coronary circulation?

Increasing blood flow is the only way to increase O$_2$ delivery in the coronary circulation because extraction is nearly maximal during resting conditions.

What is the term for the load a muscle is trying to move during stimulation?

Afterload

What is the term for days 1 to 7 of the female cycle?

Menses

What is the term for the force the ventricular muscle must generate to expel the blood into the aorta?

Afterload

What happens to the tonicity of the urine with increased ADH secretion?

The urine becomes hypertonic because of water reabsorption in the collecting duct.

What form of renal tubular reabsorption is characterized by high back leak, low affinity for substance, and absence of saturation and is surmised to be a constant percentage of a reabsorbed filtered substance?

Gradient-time system

What type of circuit is described when the total resistance is *always greater* than the sums of the individual resistors?

Series circuit

What hormone excess brings about abnormal glucose tolerance testing, impaired cardiac function, decreased body fat, increased body protein, prognathism, coarse facial features, and enlargements of the hands and feet?

Increased secretion of GH postpuberty leading to acromegaly.

What happens to V/Q ratio if a thrombus is lodged in the pulmonary artery?

The V/Q ratio **increases,** since the area is **ventilated** but **hypoperfused** as a result of the occlusion.

What hormone has the following effects: *chondrogenic* in the epiphyseal end plates of bones; *increases* AA transport for *protein synthesis*; *increases* hydroxyproline (collagen); and *increases chondroitin sulfate* synthesis?

GH, especially IGF-1. GH also *increases* the incorporation of **thymidine** in DNA synthesis and **uridine** in RNA synthesis.

True or false? Bile pigments and bile salts are reabsorbed in the gallbladder.

False

What component of an ECG is associated with the following?

    Conduction delay in the AV node

    PR interval

Ventricular depolarization	QRS complex
Atrial depolarization	P wave
Ventricular repolarization	T wave
Where is the greatest venous PO_2 in resting tissue?	Renal circulation
Near the end of pregnancy, what hormone's receptors increase in the myometrium because of elevated plasma estrogen levels?	Oxytocin
What respiratory center in the rostral pons has an inhibitory affect on the apneustic center?	Pneumotaxic center (short, fast breaths)
For what hormone do Leydig cells have receptors?	LH
What primary acid-base disturbance is cause by a *decrease in alveolar ventilation* (increasing CO_2 levels) resulting in the reaction *shifting to the right* and *increasing H^+ and HCO_3^- levels*?	Respiratory **acid**osis (summary: **high CO_2, high H^+, slightly high HCO_3^-**)
What lecithin: sphingomyelin ratio indicates lung maturity?	2.0 or greater
What is the term for the negative resting membrane potential becoming *more negative*?	Hyperpolarization (i.e., K^+ influx)

What type of resistance system (i.e., high or low) is formed when resistors are added in *parallel*?

A **low-resistance** system is formed by resistors added in parallel.

Why is hypothyroidism associated with night blindness?

Thyroid hormones are necessary for conversion of carotene to vitamin A.

What is the FiO_2 of room air?

0.21; it is a fancy way of saying 21% of the air is O_2.

Where are the lowest resting PO_2 levels in a resting individual?

Coronary circulation

What is the rate-limiting step in the production of *steroids*?

The conversion of CHO to pregnenolone via the enzyme desmolase

In the water deprivation test, does a patient with reduced urine flow have primary polydipsia or diabetes insipidus?

Primary polydipsia; patients with diabetes insipidus will continue to produce large volumes of dilute urine.

True or false? There is an inverse relationship between fat content and total body water.

True; the **greater** the fat, the **less** the total body water.

What is the role of the negative charge on the filtering membrane of the glomerular capillaries?

The negative charge **inhibits** the filtration of **protein anions**.

What cardiac reflex is characterized by stretch receptors in the right atrium, afferent and efferent limbs via the vagus nerve, and increased stretch leading to an

Bainbridge reflex

increase in heart rate via inhibition of parasympathetic stimulation?

Where in the GI tract does the reabsorption of bile salts take place?

Bile salts are actively reabsorbed in the **distal ileum.**

What three structures increase the surface area of the GI tract?

1. Plicae circularis (3 times)
2. Villi (30 times)
3. Microvilli (600 times)

Does physiologic splitting of the first heart sound occur during inspiration or expiration? Why?

Splitting of the first heart sound occurs during **inspiration** because of the **increased output** of the **right ventricle,** delaying the closure of the pulmonic valve.

How much dietary iodine is necessary to maintain normal thyroid hormone secretion?

150 mcg/day is the minimal daily intake needed. Most people ingest 500 mcg/day.

What is the central chemoreceptor's main drive for ventilation?

CSF H^+ levels, with **acidosis** being the **main central drive,** resulting in **hyperventilation** (the opposite being true with alkalosis)

What result occurs because of the negative alveolar pressure generated during inspiration?

Air flows into the respiratory system.

Corticotropin-releasing hormone promotes the synthesis and release of what prohormone?

Pro-opiomelanocortin (POMC) is cleaved into ACTH and β-lipotropin.

What happens to free hormone levels when the liver _decreases production_ and _release_ of binding proteins?

Free hormone levels remain **constant,** and the **bound hormone** level _changes_ with a decrease in binding hormones.

What type of estrogen is produced in peripheral tissues from androgens?

Estrone

What changes does more negative intrathoracic pressure cause to systemic venous return and to the pulmonary vessels?

Promotes systemic venous return into the chest and increases the caliber and volume of the pulmonary vessels

Where is renin produced?

In the JG cells of the kidney

True or false? Right-sided valves close *before* the valves on the left side of the heart.

False. Right-sided valves are the **first to open** and **last to close.**

What enzyme is associated with osteoblastic activity?

Alkaline phosphatase

What is the order of attachment of O_2 to Hgb-binding sites in the lung? Order of release from the binding sites in the tissue?

Order of attachment is site 1, 2, 3, 4, and for release is 4, 3, 2, 1.

What hormone is secreted into the plasma in response to a meal rich in protein or CHO?

Insulin

What happens to blood flow and pressure *downstream* with local arteriolar *constriction*?

With arteriolar constriction both the flow and pressure *downstream* **decrease.**

What occurs when the lower esophageal sphincter

Achalasia

fails to relax during swallowing due to abnormalities of the enteric nervous plexus?

True or false? Ungated channels are always open.

True. They have no gates, so by definition they are always open.

What component of the ANS is responsible for dilation of the blood vessels in the erectile tissue of the penis, resulting in an erection?

Parasympathetics (parasympathetics point, sympathetics shoot)

What muscle type is characterized by low ATPase activity, aerobic metabolism, myoglobin, association with endurance, and small muscle mass?

Red muscle

What happens to diastolic and systolic intervals with an *increase* in *sympathetic* activity?

Systolic interval **decreases** secondary to **increased contractility; diastolic** interval **decreases** secondary to an **increase in heart rate.**

Circulating levels of what hormone in men is responsible for the negative feedback loop to the hypothalamus and the anterior pituitary gland regulating the release of LH?

Testosterone

How are pulse pressure and compliance related?

They are **inversely proportional** to each other; as pulse pressure **increases,** compliance **decreases**.

What three substances stimulate parietal cells?

ACh, histamine, and gastrin

What two factors result in the *base* of the lung being *hyperperfused*?

Increased pulmonary arterial pressure (high perfusion) and more distensible vessels (low resistance) result in increased blood flow at the base.

True or false? Without ADH the collecting duct would be impermeable to water.

True. Without ADH **hypotonic** urine would be formed.

How does ventricular *depolarization* take place, base to apex or vice versa?

Depolarization is from apex to base and from endocardium to epicardium.

What are effects of PTH in the kidney?

PTH **increases Ca^{2+}** reabsorption in the **DCT** of the kidney and **decreases PO_4^-** reabsorption in the **PCT.**

Regarding muscle mechanics, how is passive tension produced?

It is produced by the **preload** on the muscle *prior* to contraction.

Insulin-induced hypoglycemia is the most reliable (by far not the safest) test for what hormone deficiency?

GH deficiency

In regards to *solute concentration*, how does water flow?

Water flows from a **low-solute to high-solute** concentrations.

Which extravascular chemoreceptor detects low NaCl concentrations?

Macula densa

If the AV difference is positive, is the substance extracted or produced by the organ?

A **positive** AV difference indicates that a substance is **extracted** by the organ, and a **negative** difference indicates that it is **produced** by the organ.

What is used as an index of the number of functioning carriers for a substance in active reabsorption in the kidney?

Transport maximum (Tm) occurs when all function carriers are saturated and therefore is an index of the number of functioning carriers.

Why is there a transcellular shift in K^+ levels in a diabetic patient who becomes *acidotic*?

The increased H^+ moves intracellularly and is buffered by K^+ leaving the cells, resulting in intracellular depletion and serum excess. (Intracellular hypokalemia is the reason you supplement potassium in diabetic ketoacidosis, even though the serum levels are elevated.)

True or false? COMT is *not* found in smooth muscle, liver, and the kidneys.

False. That is precisely where COMT is found; it is *not found* in **adrenergic nerve** terminals.

What somatomedin serves as a 24-hour marker of GH secretion?

IGF-1 (somatomedin C)

What receptor is in the smooth muscle cells of the small bronchi, is stimulated during inflation, and inhibits inspiration?

Stretch receptors prevent overdistension of the lungs during inspiration.

True or false? Thyroid hormones are necessary for normal menstrual cycles.

True. They are also necessary for normal brain maturation.

What component of the cardiovascular system has the largest blood volume? Second largest blood volume?

The **systemic veins** have the **largest** blood volume, and the **pulmonary veins** have the **second** largest blood volume in the cardiovascular system. They represent the reservoirs of circulation.

Serum concentration of what substance is used as a clinical measure of a patient's GFR?

Creatinine

Where does CHO digestion begin?

In the mouth with salivary α-amylase (ptyalin)

How does the sympathetic nervous system affect insulin secretion?

It **decreases** insulin secretion.

How does *cell diameter* affect the conduction velocity of an action potential?

The **greater** the cell diameter, the **greater** the conduction velocity.

6

Pharmacology

True or false?
Hyperkalemia _increases_ the effect of digoxin.

False. hyperkalemia decreases digoxin's activity, while hypokalemia, hypomagnesemia, and hypercalcemia all increase digoxin toxicity.

Which antispasmodic blocks the release of Ca^{2+} from the SR and is used in the treatment of malignant hyperthermia?

Dantrolene

Which _overdose_ carries a higher mortality rate, that of benzodiazepines or barbiturates?

Barbiturate overdose and **benzodiazepine withdrawal** carry the highest mortality rates.

What antiviral agent is used in the treatment of drug-induced Parkinson's disease?

Amantadine

Are the following responses associated with histamines H_1 or H_2 receptor activation?

Edema	H_1
Gastric acid secretion	H_2
SA nodal activity	H_2
Pain and pruritus	H_1
Bronchial smooth muscle activity	H_1

Inotropic action and automaticity	H_2
True or false? The lack of dopamine production in the substantia nigra leads to the extrapyramidal dysfunction, characteristically seen in patients with Parkinson's disease.	True. The lack of dopamine leads to an excess of ACh, hence extrapyramidal dysfunction.
Which PG maintains patency of the ductus arteriosus and is used in the treatment of primary pulmonary HTN?	PGI_2
Which CNS ACh receptor or receptors are excitatory? Inhibitory?	M_1 and nicotinic receptors are excitatory in the CNS and M_2 receptor is inhibitory.
True or false? β₂-Adrenergic agents are used in the management of an *acute* asthmatic attack.	True. They are useful in the **early-phase** response to an asthmatic attack.
Do local anesthetics bind to the activated or inactivated sodium channels?	Inactivated
What is the DOC for treating Tourette syndrome?	Pimozide
What mosquito is responsible for the transmission of malaria?	*Anopheles* mosquito
What enzyme is inhibited by disulfiram?	Acetaldehyde dehydrogenase

Which diuretic is used as an adrenal steroid antagonist?

Spironolactone

What drug is given transdermally for chronic pain but can cause chest wall rigidity if given IV?

Fentanyl

What is the drug of choice for penicillin-resistant gonococcal infections?

Spectinomycin

What is the DOC for treating torsade de pointes?

Magnesium

Is heparin contraindicated in pregnancy?

No. Heparin is safe in pregnancy, but warfarin is contraindicated in pregnancy because of its ability to cross the placenta.

What oral antifungal agent is used to treat dermatophyte infections by disrupting microtubule structure and depositing keratin?

Griseofulvin

Which anticonvulsant can cause teratogenic craniofacial abnormalities and spina bifida?

Carbamazepine

What are the three β-lactamase inhibitors?

1. Clavulanic acid
2. Sulbactam
3. Tazobactam

Which anticonvulsant used in the treatment of bipolar disorder is refractory to lithium?

Carbamazepine

Are antineoplastic agents that work on actively proliferating cells schedule or dose dependent?

Schedule dependent; antineoplastic agents that work on nonproliferating cells are dose dependent.

Which class of diuretics is used to treat metabolic acidosis, acute mountain sicknesses, and glaucoma and to aid in the elimination of acidic drug overdoses?

Carbonic anhydrase inhibitors (acetazolamide and dorzolamide)

What estrogen receptor agonist in bone is used in the treatment and prevention of osteoporosis?

Raloxifene

Which tetracycline is used in the treatment of SIADH?

Demeclocycline

How is the eye affected by use of opioids?

With opioid use the pupils become pinpoint (miosis) because of increased cholinergic activity.

Name the antimicrobial agent whose major side effect is listed.

Grey baby syndrome	Chloramphenicol
CN VIII damage (vestibulotoxic)	Aminoglycosides
Teratogenicity	Metronidazole
Cholestatic hepatitis	Erythromycin
Hemolytic anemia	Nitrofurantoin
Dental staining in children	Tetracycline
Altered folate metabolism	Trimethoprim
Auditory toxicity	Vancomycin
Cartilage abnormalities	Quinolones

What are the two side effects of opioids to which the user will not develop tolerance?

Constipation and miosis

Which anticonvulsant is also used in the treatment of bipolar disorder and for migraine headaches?

Valproic acid

What antitubercular agent causes loss of red-green visual discrimination?

Ethambutol

Name the insulin preparation based on the peak effect and duration of action.

Peak, 8 to 16 hours; duration, 24 to 36 hours

Ultralente

Peak, 0.5 to 3 hours; duration, 5 to 7 hours

Regular insulin

Peak, 8 to 12 hours; duration, 18 to 24 hours

Lente or NPH insulin (neutral protamine Hagedorn insulin)

Peak, 0.3 to 2 hours; duration, 3 to 4 hours

Lispro insulin

Is digoxin or digitoxin *renally* eliminated?

Digoxin is renally eliminated; digitoxin is hepatically eliminated.

What is the DOC for steroid-induced osteoporosis?

Alendronate

What are the first signs of overdose from phenobarbitals?

Nystagmus and ataxia

How are lipid solubility and potency related for inhaled anesthetics? How do they affect onset and recovery?

Inhaled anesthetics with **low** lipid solubility have **low** potency (directly related), so they have **rapid** induction and **rapid** recovery; vice versa for drugs with high lipid solubility.

What α_1-agonist, not inactivated by COMT, is used as a decongestant and for treatment of paroxysmal atrial tachycardia?

Phenylephrine

Which laxative is used in the treatment of *hepatic encephalopathy*?

Lactulose

Are hydrolysis, oxidation, and reduction phase I or II biotransformations?

Phase I

What β-blocker is also an α-blocker?

Labetalol

What agent is used IM to treat acute dystonias?

Diphenhydramine

True or false? Anaerobes are resistant to the effects of aminoglycosides.

True. Aminoglycosides use O_2-dependent uptake and therefore are ineffective for treatment of anaerobic infections.

What two β-blockers decrease serum lipids?

Pindolol and acebutolol

If a drug is *ionized*, is it water or lipid soluble? Can it cross a biomembrane?

Ionized drugs are **water soluble,** and since only lipid-soluble drugs can cross biomembranes, an ionized drug **cannot** cross them without the help of a carrier.

What are the longest-acting and shortest-acting benzodiazepines?

Diazepam is longest acting and **midazolam** is shortest acting.

What is the DOC for severe infections with *Sporothrix*, *Mucor*, *Histoplasma*, *Cryptococcus*, *Candida*, and *Aspergillus*?

Amphotericin B

What neurotransmitter is *presynaptically* inhibited by reserpine and guanethidine?

NE

Which two cephalosporins cross the blood-brain barrier?

Cefuroxime and cefaclor

What agent, in combination with a MAOI inhibitor, can cause hypertensive crisis?

Tyramine

True or false? Cocaine-induced coronary ischemia should not be treated with β-blockers.

True. β-Blockade would result in unopposed α-adrenergic stimulation and worsen the patient's symptoms. Calcium channel blockers are the way to go.

What antimuscarinic is used as an inhalant for asthma?

Ipratropium

What two forms of insulin, if mixed together, precipitate zinc?

Lente insulin and either NPH or protamine zinc insulin (PZI)

What androgen receptor blocker is used in the treatment of prostatic cancer?

Flutamide

What are the first signs of phenobarbital overdose?

Nystagmus and ataxia

Which virus is treated with the monoclonal antibody palivizumab?

RSV

Which medication used in the treatment of bipolar disorder decreases the release of T_4 from the thyroid gland?	Lithium
Which class of antiarrhythmics are potassium channel blockers?	Class III
Which muscarinic receptor uses a decrease in adenyl cyclase as its second messenger?	M_2
What antiepileptic agent has SIADH as a side effect?	Carbamazepine
What is the only anesthetic that causes cardiovascular stimulation?	Ketamine
Which bacteriostatic drug whose major side effect is the lepra reaction inhibits folic acid synthesis?	Dapsone
What form of antimicrobial therapy is best for an immunocompromised patient?	Bactericidal
Which direct-acting vasodilator is associated with SLE-like syndrome in slow acetylators?	Hydralazine
What class of heparin is active against factor Xa and has no effect on PT or PT?	Low molecular weight heparin (LMWH)
What is the DOC for coccidioidomycosis?	Fluconazole

What three cephalosporins have good penetration against *Bacteroides fragilis*?

1. Cefotetan
2. Cefoxitin
3. Ceftizoxime

Which form of alcohol toxicity results in ocular damage?

Methanol

What immunosuppressive agent is converted to 6-mercaptopurine?

Azathioprine

Which size nerve fibers (small or large diameter) are more sensitive to local anesthetic blockade?

Nerve fibers with **small diameter** and **high firing rates** are **most sensitive** to local blockade.

What enzyme is inhibited by trimethoprim?

Dihydrofolate reductase

What are the two absolute requirements for the cytochrome P450 enzyme system?

NADPH and molecular O_2

What three PGs are potent platelet aggregators?

PGE_1, PGI_2 (most potent), and TXA_2

A depressive patient who is taking paroxetine goes to the ER with pain and is given meperidine. Shortly afterward she develops diaphoresis, myoclonus, muscle rigidity, hyperthermia, and seizures. What is your diagnosis?

Serotonergic crisis may be precipitated when an SSRI is mixed with MAOIs, TCADs, dextromethorphan, and meperidine. Treat it with cyproheptadine.

What class of drugs is used in the treatment of demineralization of the bone?

Bisphosphonates

What is the only class of diuretics to retain Cl⁻ used in the short-term treatment of glaucoma and of acute mountain sickness?	Acetazolamide
True or false? All aluminum-containing antacids can cause hypophosphatemia.	True. Aluminum reacts with PO_4^-, resulting in $AlPO_4$, an insoluble compound that cannot be absorbed.
What TCAD causes sudden cardiac death in children?	Desipramine
What two β₂-agonists are used to produce bronchodilation?	Metaproterenol and albuterol
What *IV-only* agent inhibits water reabsorption in the PCTs and is used to treat increased intracranial pressure, increased intraocular pressure, and acute renal failure?	Mannitol
What cell type do cromolyn and nedocromil affect for prophylactic management of asthma via blockade?	They prevent mast cell degranulation.
What two β₂-agonists cause myometrial relaxation?	Ritodrine and terbutaline
Where in the spinal cord are the presynaptic opioid receptors?	In the dorsal horn of the spinal cord on the primary afferent neurons
What thrombolytic agent is derived from β-hemolytic streptococci, is antigenic, and produces depletion of	Streptokinase

circulating fibrinogen, plasminogen, and factors V and VII?

What antifungal agent is used to treat dermatophyte infections by inhibiting squalene epoxidase? Terbinafine

Which class of antihypertensives produces angioedema, hyperkalemia, and a dry cough? ACE inhibitors (the -pril agents)

Which medication requires an *acidic gastric pH* for activation to form a protective gel-like coating over ulcers and GI epithelium? Sucralfate

Of what serotonin receptor is sumatriptan an agonist? 5HT1D

A patient with a history of epilepsy goes to the ER with sedation, gait ataxia, diplopia, and vertical nystagmus. Which anticonvulsant overdose resulted in the patient's symptoms? Phenytoin

What are the five penicillinase-resistant penicillins?
1. **C**loxacillin
2. **O**xacillin
3. **N**afcillin
4. **D**icloxacillin
5. **M**ethicillin
(CONDM)

Which aminoglycoside is the DOC for tularemia and the bubonic plague? Streptomycin

Is the following description characteristic of competitive or noncompetitive antagonists: parallel shift to the right on a dose-response curve, complete reversibility with increase of the dose of the agonist drug, and capacity to decrease the potency of the agonist drug?

Competitive antagonist

True or false? Progestins are used in combination with estrogens to decrease the risk of endometrial cancer.

True

What neuroleptic agent causes agranulocytosis but does not induce tardive dyskinesia?

Clozapine

What two factors influence low oral bioavailability?

First-pass metabolism and acid lability

What is the only site in the body that uses M_1 receptors?

The stomach

What vitamin is a cofactor of aromatic AACD and decreases the efficacy of L-dopa if used concomitantly?

Vitamin B_6 (pyridoxine)

True or false? Acetaminophen has analgesic and antipyretic activities but *lacks* anti-inflammatory effects.

True

What happens to plasma concentration of a drug if there is a large volume of distribution?

The **larger** the **volume of distribution,** the **lower** the **plasma concentration** of a drug.

Why should opioid analgesics be avoided for patients with head trauma?

Opioids cause cerebral vasodilation and can result in **increased intracerebral pressure.**

What is the drug of choice in the treatment of the lepra reaction?

Clofazimine

What two drugs, when mixed, can lead to malignant hyperthermia?

Succinylcholine and halothane (Treatment is with dantrolene.)

What three β-blockers are used in the treatment of glaucoma?

1. Propranolol
2. Timolol
3. Carteolol

What is the neurotransmitter at the κ-receptor?

Dynorphin

True or false? Succinylcholine is a nicotinic receptor agonist.

True

What is the drug of choice for hypertensive patients with a decreased renal function?

α-Methyldopa (Guanabenz or clonidine is also used.)

What is the volume of distribution (increased or decreased) of a drug when a large percentage is protein bound?

Volume of distribution is **decreased** when a large percentage of drug is protein bound.

What antihistamine is used in the treatment of serotonergic crisis?

Cyproheptadine

What is the drug of choice for early Parkinson's disease?

Selegiline

What is the site of action of the following?

    Osmotic diuretics

The entire tubule barring the thick ascending limb

    Loop diuretics

Ascending limb

    Thiazide diuretics

Early distal tubule

    K^+-sparing diuretics

Early collecting duct

    Aldosterone antagonists

Distal convoluted tubules

What hematologic malignancy is treated with the monoclonal antibody rituximab?

Non-Hodgkin lymphoma

Which sodium channel blocker is used to treat *lithium-induced diabetes insipidus*?

Amiloride

Which two antipsychotic drugs create a high risk for developing EPS side effects?

Haloperidol and fluphenazine (but use of any high-potency phenothiazine runs the risk of EPS)

Could an overdose with either zolpidem or zaleplon be reversed with flumazenil?

Yes, because they both activate the BZ_1-receptors, which can be reversed by flumazenil.

What drug blocks intragranular uptake of NE?

Reserpine

True or false? Antimicrobial agents that slow bacterial growth are bactericidal.

False. Bacteriocidals kill; bacteriostatics slow growth.

Which antihyperlipidemic agent would you not prescribe for a patient with a history of *gout* or *PUD*?

Nicotinic acid, because its side effects include hyperuricemia and exacerbation of ulcers.

What inhibitor of microtubule synthesis is the drug of choice for whipworm and pinworm?

Mebendazole

What antiviral agents inhibit neuraminidases of influenza A and B?

Zanamivir and oseltamivir

What three cephalosporins inhibit vitamin K–dependent factors?

Cefamandole, cefoperazone, and moxalactam

Which direct-acting vasodilator is used clinically to treat hypertensive emergencies, insulinomas, and as a uterine smooth muscle relaxant?

Diazoxide

Which leukotriene—LTA4, LTB4, LTC4, or LTD4—is *not* associated with anaphylaxis and bronchoconstriction?

LTB4

What neuroleptic agent causes retinal deposits, hypotension, and torsades de pointes?

Thioridazine

What oral hypoglycemic agent inhibits α-glucosidase in the brush border of the small intestine?

Acarbose

What enzyme is inhibited by sulfonamides?

Dihydropteroate synthetase

What is the most important determinant of drug potency?

The affinity of the drug for its receptor

True or false? Estrogen use increases the risk of developing ovarian cancer.

False. Risk of breast and endometrial cancer but not ovarian cancer increases with the use of estrogen.

Which sedative–hypnotic is contraindicated for patients taking warfarin?

Chloral hydrate

What mixed α-antagonists are used for patients with pheochromocytoma?

Phentolamine and phenoxybenzamine

What are the four types of signaling mechanisms?

1. Intracellular receptors
2. Membrane receptors
3. Enzymes
4. Intracellular effectors

The dose of which second-generation sulfonylurea agent must be decreased for patients with hepatic dysfunction?

The dose of **glipizide** must be decreased in hepatic dysfunction. Glyburide's dose must be decreased in renal dysfunction.

Which nicotinic receptor antagonist causes hypotension and is associated with malignant hyperthermia?

d-Tubocurarine

What transient deficiency may result in a hypercoagulable state if warfarin is given alone?

Transient **protein C deficiency,** because of its relatively short half-life, may result if warfarin is instituted alone.

What component of the vascular system is most sensitive to the effects of calcium channel blockers?

Arterioles

What drug blocks glucose uptake, leading to decreased formation of ATP and resulting in immobilization of the parasite?

Albendazole

What is the site of action for carbonic anhydrase inhibitors?

Proximal tubule

What phase of the cell cycle are the following antineoplastic agents specific for?

Bleomycin	G2 phase
Cytarabine	S phase
Vinblastine	Mitosis
Alkylating agents	G0 phase
Paclitaxel	Mitosis
Vincristine	Mitosis
6-Thioguanine	S phase
6-Mercaptopurine	S phase
Dacarbazine	G0 phase
Hydroxyurea	S phase
Cisplatin	G0 phase
Nitrosoureas	G0 phase

Inhibition of peripheral COMT, allowing increased CNS availability of L-dopa, is accomplished by what two agents?

Tolcapone and entacapone

What medication is a *PGE₁ analog* that results in increased secretions of mucus and HCO₃⁻ in the GI tract?

Misoprostol

Is there a difference between mathematical and clinical steady states? If so, what are their values (half-lives)?

There is a difference; it takes about 7 to 8 half-lives to reach mathematical steady state and **4 to 5 half-lives** to reach **clinical steady state**.

True or false? At high doses aspirin has uricosuric properties.

True. At **high doses** ASA **decreases** uric acid **reabsorption** in the renal tubules, resulting in uricosuric actions. At **low doses** ASA **decreases** tubular **secretion** of uric acid, leading to hyperuricemia.

What antiviral agent is used to treat RSV, influenza A and B, Lassa fever, and hantavirus and as an adjunct to IFN-α in hepatitis C?

Ribavirin

Which aminoglycoside is used only topically because it is too toxic for systemic use?

Neomycin

Which class of antiarrhythmics blocks sodium channels?

Class 1 (1A, 1B, and 1C)

What form of penicillin is used in the treatment of life-threatening illnesses?

Penicillin G (benzylpenicillin)

What is the DOC for esophageal candidiasis?

Fluconazole

True or false? Flumazenil is used in the treatment of barbiturate overdose.

False. Flumazenil is unable to block the effects of barbiturates.

Which three aminoglycosides have vestibular toxicity?

1. Streptomycin
2. Gentamicin
3. Tobramycin

What is the term for the amount of a drug that is needed to produce the desired effect?

Potency

What agent used in the treatment of BPH and baldness is a 5-α-reductase inhibitor?

Finasteride

What β-blocker is also a membrane stabilizer?

Propranolol

Name one of the ADP receptor antagonists used in patients who are post-MI, have had TIAs, have unstable angina, and are allergic to ASA?

Ticlopidine or clopidogrel

What is the treatment for nephrogenic diabetes insipidus induced by lithium?

Amiloride

Which calcium channel blocker is used to treat *subarachnoid hemorrhages* by preventing posthemorrhagic vasospasms?

Nimodipine

What two drugs inhibit the release of neurotransmitters from storage granules?

Guanethidine and bretylium

What is the DOC for hyperprolactinemia?

Pergolide

True or false? The faster the rate of absorption, the smaller the time of maximum concentration (T_{max}) and the maximum concentration (C_{max}).

False. The **faster** the rate of absorption, the **smaller the T_{max} and larger the C_{max}** (bioinequivalence). The slower the rate of absorption, the larger the T_{max} and smaller the C_{max}.

What tetracycline is associated with hepatotoxicity?

Chlortetracycline

What is the term for how well a drug produces its desired response?

Efficacy

What drug, if given during pregnancy, would cause the uterus to exhibit signs of progesterone withdrawal and induce an abortion?

RU 486

Is allopurinol used in the *acute* treatment of gout?

No, it is used in *chronic* treatment of gout to decrease the uric acid pools in the body.

What three cephalosporins can produce disulfiram-like reactions?

1. Cefamandole
2. Cefoperazone
3. Moxalactam

What is the physiologic basis for the actions of birth control pills?

They block the midcycle surge of LH.

When a drug is administered orally and enters into portal circulation, it undergoes hepatic metabolism. What is the name of this effect?

First-pass effect

Which thrombolytic agent, activated in the presence of fibrin, is manufactured by recombinant DNA process?

Alteplase

Which benzodiazepine is most commonly used IV in conscious sedation protocols?

Midazolam

What is the drug of choice for threadworm, trichinosis, and larva migrans?

Thiabendazole

Can you tell which drug is more toxic based on therapeutic indices alone?

No, therapeutic indices can tell which drug is **safer,** not more toxic.

What blood disorder is a side effect of metformin?

Megaloblastic anemia (decreased absorption of vitamin B_{12} and folic acid)

A schizophrenic patient who is taking haloperidol is brought to your ER with muscle rigidity, a temperature of 104°F, altered mental status, and hypotension. What is your diagnosis and what is the treatment?

Neuroleptic malignant syndrome is a potentially life-threatening condition which is treated with symptomatic support, **bromocriptine,** and **dantrolene.**

Which α-blocking agent is used to treat refractory hypertension and baldness?

Minoxidil (orally and topically, respectively!)

What components of the coagulation cascade are affected by estrogen?

Estrogen can result in a hypercoagulable state because of the decrease in AT III and increase in factors II, VII, IX, and X.

What class of antimicrobial agents should be avoided in patients with a history of GPDH deficiency?

Sulfonamides

What enzyme of cholesterol synthesis is inhibited by the statins?

HMG-CoA reductase

What bactericidal agents are resistant to β-lactamases and are used to treat in-hospital life-threatening infections?

Imipenem and meropenem

What adrenergic receptors use inositol triphosphate (IP$_3$) and diacylglycerol (DAG) for their second messenger system?

α_1-Receptors

True or false? Dopamine antagonists at the D2A receptor have the capacity to induce pseudoparkinsonism.

True

What two PGs are used to induce labor?

PGE$_2$ and PGF$_{2\alpha}$

How are drugs that are excreted via the biliary system resorbed by the GI tract?

Enterohepatic cycling

Which drugs bind to the 30S ribosomal subunit and interfere with the initiation complex, causing a misreading of mRNA?

Aminoglycosides

What antiviral agent blocks the attachment and penetration of influenza A virus?

Amantadine

What is the antidote for organophosphate ingestion?

Atropine and 2-PAM (pralidoxime)

Which antihypertensive class is used to help stop the progression of microalbuminuria?

ACE inhibitors (-pril)

What class of drugs are the DOCs for peptic ulcer disease, Zollinger-Ellison syndrome, and gastroesophageal reflux disease?	Proton pump inhibitors
What bacteriostatic agent's side effect profile includes grey baby syndrome and aplastic anemia?	Chloramphenicol
Inhibition of peripheral aromatic AADC and increased CNS availability of L-dopa are results of what drug used in the treatment of Parkinson's disease?	Carbidopa and benserazide

What type of drug elimination is characterized by the following?

Elimination *independent* of plasma concentration; constant *amount* eliminated per unit time; no fixed half-life	Zero-order elimination
Elimination *directly proportional* to plasma level; constant *fraction* eliminated per unit time; fixed half-life	First-order elimination
True or false? NSAIDs have analgesic, antipyretic, anti-inflammatory, and antiplatelet activities.	True
True or false? Tetracyclines are bactericidal.	False. They are bacteriostatic.

What class 1A antiarrhythmic agent has SLE-like syndrome side effect in slow acetylators?	Procainamide
What is the major pulmonary side effect of μ-activators?	Respiratory depression
What neuroleptic agent is also considered to be an antihistamine?	Risperidone
What form of penicillin is stable in acid environments?	Penicillin V
What is the term for the proportion of a drug that reaches systemic circulation?	Bioavailability
What two drugs block dopa-decarboxylase in the periphery to decrease the conversion of L-dopa to dopamine?	Carbidopa and benserazide
What is the DOC for bipolar disorder?	Lithium
True or false? If a mother delivers a Rho-positive baby, she should receive Rho-immunoglobulin.	True if she is Rho-negative; false if she is Rho-positive
True or false? Both GABA and glutamic acid are excitatory neurotransmitters in the CNS.	False. Glutamic acid is excitatory, but GABA is inhibitory.
What is the drug of choice for asymptomatic meningitis carriers?	Rifampin

What drug is used to differentiate a cholinergic crisis from myasthenia gravis?

Edrophonium

What class of antianginal activates the NO pathway to produce endothelial vasodilation?

Nitrates

What selective Cox-2 inhibitor should be avoided in patients with a history of sulfonamide allergy?

Celecoxib

What is the DOC for blastomycoses and sporotrichoses?

Itraconazole

What are the two most important features in the diagnosis of malaria?

Splenomegaly and anemia (with a high index of suspicion)

Name the three benzodiazepines that are *not* metabolized by the cytochrome P450 enzyme system.

Oxazepam, **t**emazepam, and lorazepam (**OTL, O**utside **T**he **L**iver)

What drug is an M_1-specific antispasmodic?

Pirenzepine

Which centrally acting α_2-adrenergic agonist is safe for use in renal dysfunction and in HTN during pregnancy?

Methyldopa

What is the monoamine oxidase B (MAOB) inhibitor?

Selegiline

What antitubercular agent causes a red-orange tinge to tears and urine?

Rifampin

What two classes of drugs can cause schizoid behavior?

Glucocorticoids and amphetamines

What tetracycline is associated with vestibular toxicity?

Minocycline

What is the most potent NMJ blocker and also has no cardiovascular side effects?

Doxacurium

What two receptors in the chemoreceptor trigger zone lead to vomiting when stimulated?

D2 and 5HT3 receptors

Which group of antihypertensive agents best decreases left ventricular hypertrophy?

Thiazide diuretics

What area of the brain is linked to emotion and movement?

Mesolimbic system

Why are clozapine and olanzapine unlikely to result in EPS effects?

Because they do not block D2A receptors, they are antagonists of 5HT2 receptors.

What class of pharmaceuticals are inactive until they are metabolized to their active products?

Prodrugs

True or false? You would not prescribe probenecid for a patient with gout who is an *overexcretor of uric acid.*

True. Probenecid can precipitate uric acid crystals in the kidney if the patient is an overexcretor of urate.

True or false? Dopamine *antagonists* are antiemetic.

True. They block the dopamine receptors in the chemoreceptor trigger zone.

What bactericidal agent is the DOC for MRSA, enterococci, and *Clostridium difficile?*

Vancomycin

True or false? β-Blockers are contraindicated in patients who *present to the hospital* with CHF.

True. β-Blockers are a component of CHF regimen for stable patients, not those who are decompensated. (This means you discharge a patient from the hospital with a prescription for a β-blocker; you don't start β-blockers when the patient is admitted.)

True or false? Fluoroquinolones are bactericidal.

True. They inhibit DNA gyrase (topo II).

What antiviral agent for ganciclovir-resistant infections has limited utility because of its nephrotoxic side effect?

Foscarnet

What oral hypoglycemic agent stimulates pancreatic β-cell release of insulin and is given just prior to meals because of its short half-life?

Repaglinide

True or false? There is no absorption of an IV-administered drug.

True. No loss of drug and no absorption if a drug is given IV.

What hypothesis states that an antineoplastic agent kills a fixed *percentage* of tumor cells, not a fixed number?

Log-kill hypothesis (follows first order kinetics)

What is the only local anesthetic to produce vasoconstriction?	Cocaine
Which agent used in the treatment of asthma is a selective inhibitor of the lipoxygenase pathway?	Zileuton
What is the only diuretic that works on the blood side of the nephron?	Spironolactone (binds to aldosterone receptors)
Do you monitor heparin's therapeutic levels by PT or PTT?	Heparin, intrinsic pathway, PTT; warfarin, extrinsic pathway, PT (mnemonic: hPeT, wPiTT)
What is the only neuroleptic that does not cause an increase in weight or appetite?	Molindone
What α_1-agonist is used to treat paroxysmal atrial tachycardia with hypotension?	Metaraminol (α_1, β_1)
What antiarrhythmic agent is the DOC for treating and diagnosing PSVT and AV nodal arrhythmias?	Adenosine (it is an excellent agent to use in emergencies because its half-life is 30 seconds)
What phosphodiesterase inhibitor is used *IV* in the management of *status asthmaticus*?	Aminophylline
Which nicotinic receptor antagonist is inactivated to laudanosine?	Atracurium
What α_2-antagonist is used to treat impotence and postural hypotension?	Yohimbine

What drug of choice for ascaris causes neuromuscular blockade of the worm?

Pyrantel pamoate

Testing of a drug in a small group of volunteers without the disease is a component of which phase of clinical drug testing?

Phase 1

Which antimicrobial class may cause tooth enamel dysplasia and decreased bone growth in children?

Tetracycline

What antifungal agent is used in the treatment of androgen receptor–positive cancers?

Ketoconazole

What MAOI does not cause a hypertensive crisis?

Selegiline

Which penicillin can cause interstitial nephritis?

Methicillin

Is hirsutism a side effect of estrogen or progestin therapy?

Progestin

Which potassium-sparing drug is an *aldosterone receptor antagonist*?

Spironolactone

What are the three signs of morphine overdose?

1. Pinpoint pupils
2. Decreased respiratory rate
3. Coma

Which anticonvulsant is used in the treatment of bipolar disorder and neuropathic pain?

Gabapentin

True or false? Metformin is contraindicated in obese patients because of weight gain as its side effect.

False. Metformin does not have weight gain as a potential side effect (unlike sulfonylureas).

What is the DOC for the treatment of the *late phase* response in an asthmatic attack?

Corticosteroid

If you double the infusion rate of a drug, how long will it take to reach steady state?

Regardless of the rate of infusion, it takes 4 to 5 half-lives to reach steady state.

What is the neurotransmitter at the μ-receptor?

β-Endorphin

What is the DOC for the following protozoal infections?

    Amebiasis

Metronidazole

    Leishmaniasis

Stibogluconate

    ***Pneumocystis carinii* pneumonia**

Trimethoprim/sulfamethoxazole (TMP-SMX)

    Giardiasis

Metronidazole

    Trichomoniasis

Metronidazole

What hematologic agent is used in the treatment of intermittent claudication because it decreases blood viscosity and increases RBC membrane flexibility and stability?

Pentoxifylline

What enzyme system is the most common form of phase II biotransformation?	Glucuronidation
In what three areas of the body are sympathetics the predominant tone?	1. Sweat glands 2. Arterioles 3. Veins
What is the only antifungal agent to penetrate CSF?	Fluconazole
Which class of antiarrhythmics are β-blockers?	Class II
What three cephalosporins are eliminated via biliary mechanisms?	1. Cefamandole 2. Cefoperazone 3. Ceftriaxone
Which centrally acting α₂-adrenergic agonist is used in the treatment protocol of opioid withdrawal?	Clonidine
What is the name of the monoclonal antibody used in the treatment of Crohn disease and rheumatoid arthritis?	Infliximab
Which macrolide is used in the treatment of gastroparesis?	Erythromycin
What syndrome is characterized by the triad of renal tubular acidosis, nephrosis, and amino aciduria?	Fanconi-like syndrome
In what area of the brain can an excess of dopamine lead to psychotic symptoms?	Mesocortical area

Name five causes for zero-order metabolism.

1. Sustained release
2. IV drip
3. Phenytoin
4. Alcohol
5. Aspirin toxicity

What antitubercular agent requires vitamin B$_6$ supplementation?

Isoniazid

Which antihistamine is one of the DOCs for treatment of vertigo?

Meclizine

What is the DOC for treating *Entamoeba histolytica*, *Giardia*, *Trichomonas*, *Bacillus fragilis*, and *Clostridium difficile* infections?

Metronidazole

Which class of antihypertensives is used in the treatment of BPH?

α-Blockers (-zosins)

Which macrolide is given as 1200 mg/week for the prophylaxis of *Mycobacterium avium-intracellulare* complex?

Azithromycin

What is the drug of choice, which inhibits oxidative phosphorylation in cestodes, for taeniasis?

Niclosamide

Which class of antihyperlipidemics would you avoid for a patient with elevated triglyceride levels?

Bile acid sequestrants (cholestyramine and colestipol) increase VLDL and triglyceride levels; therefore, they are not used if a patient has hypertriglyceridemia.

True or false? Ergotamines, because of their vasodilation action, are

False. Ergotamines are used in the treatment of migraines for their **vasoconstrictive** action in the cerebral

used in the treatment of migraines.

circulation.

Is DM a contraindication to use of a β-blocker in a patient who is having an MI?

Absolutely not. Diabetics who are given a β-blocker for an acute chest syndrome have significantly better outcomes than those who do not.

What β$_2$-agonist is used as a prophylactic agent in the treatment of asthma?

Salmeterol

What hormone can be affected by dopamine release in the tuberoinfundibular pathway?

In the tuberoinfundibular pathway, dopamine release will **decrease prolactin** release, which is why dopamine agonists are used in the treatment of hyperprolactinemic states.

What determines the plasma level at steady state?

The rate of infusion

What enzyme is inhibited by propylthiouracil (PTU)?

5′ deiodinase

What is the DOC for CMV retinitis?

Ganciclovir

What agent antagonizes the effects of heparin?

Protamine sulfate

What antihypertensive agent produces cyanide and thiocyanate as byproducts?

Nitroprusside

What is the DOC for *β-blocker-induced* bronchospasms?

Ipratropium

What is the only neuroleptic agent that does not cause hyperprolactinemia?

Clozapine

True or false?
Gynecomastia is a side
effect of cimetidine.

True. Cimetidine can decrease androgen production and lead to gynecomastia.

What three drugs are
associated with SLE-like
syndrome in slow
acetylators?

Hydralazine, isoniazid, and procainamide (HIP)

What is the drug of choice
for filariasis and
onchocerciasis?

Diethylcarbamazine

What aminoglycoside
causes disruption of CN I?

Streptomycin

Which anticonvulsant
causes gingival hyperplasia?

Phenytoin (cyclosporine and nifedipine also result in gingival hyperplasia)

What is the only NSAID
that causes *irreversible*
inhibition of the
cyclooxygenase pathway?

ASA

What antifungal agent is
activated by fungal
cytosine deaminase to form
5-FU?

Flucytosine

***Irreversible* ototoxicity is**
associated with which loop
diuretic?

Ethacrynic acid

What competitive estrogen
receptor antagonist is used
in the treatment of breast
cancer?

Tamoxifen

Which tetracycline is
used to treat prostatitis
because it concentrates
strongly in prostatic fluid?

Doxycycline

True or false? Dopamine is an excitatory neurotransmitter in the CNS.

False. Dopamine is an inhibitory neurotransmitter in the CNS.

What oral hypoglycemic agent should be used with caution in patients with CHF because it causes lactic acidosis?

Metformin

Which phase of clinical drug testing includes postmarket reporting of adverse reactions?

Phase 4

Which prophylactic asthmatic agent is an antagonist of LTD4?

Zafirlukast

What are the three C's of a TCAD overdose?

Coma, convulsions, and cardiotoxicity

What is the neurotransmitter at the δ-receptor?

Enkephalin

What body fluid preferentially breaks down esters?

Blood

What are the two broad-spectrum penicillins?

Ampicillin and amoxicillin

What are the three components to the asthma triad?

Nasal polyps, rhinitis, and ASA hypersensitivity

Which class of antiarrhythmics are calcium channel blockers?

Class IV

What are the glycoprotein receptors that platelets and fibrinogen cross-link to when forming a thrombus?	GP IIb and IIIa receptors
Which IV agent has the lowest incidence of postoperative emesis and has the fastest rate of recovery?	Propofol
Are two different receptors with two different agonists characteristic of pharmacologic or physiologic antagonism?	Physiologic antagonism
What GnRH analog is used as a repository form of treatment in prostatic cancer?	Leuprolide
Which antimicrobial agent is used with pyrimethamine to treat toxoplasmosis?	Clindamycin
What is the DOC for trigeminal neuralgia?	Carbamazepine
What drug that penetrates the blood-brain barrier is found in asthma preparations and used as a nasal decongestant?	Ephedrine
What is the term for drug removal per unit of time in a given volume of blood?	Clearance
Which two tetracyclines have the highest plasma binding?	Doxycycline and minocycline

What do the following values indicate?

ED_{50}

Effective dose for 50% of drug takers (median effective dose)

TD_{50}

Toxic dose for 50% of drug takers (median toxic dose)

LD_{50}

Lethal dose for 50% of drug takers (median lethal dose)

Do agents used in the treatment of Parkinson's disease that decrease ACh function have little effect on reducing tremors and rigidity?

Agents that decrease ACh function reduce tremors and rigidity, not bradykinesias.

A patient goes to the ER with signs and symptoms of biliary colic. Which opioid analgesic do you choose?

Spasms of the uterus, bladder, and the biliary tree occur with all of the opioids except **meperidine.**

What form of oxidation takes place with the addition of a *water molecule* and breakage of bonds?

Hydrolysis

7   Pathology

What is the term for an abnormal amount of collagen type III that produces a large bulging scar, seen primarily in blacks?

Keloid

True or false? Klinefelter syndrome cannot be diagnosed until puberty.

True

What form of sunlight is the most carcinogenic?

Ultraviolet B (UVB) sunlight

What renal pathology involves uniform thickening of the glomerular capillary wall, granular appearance under the microscope, and effacement of foot processes?

MGN

What enveloped RNA retrovirus infects CD4 T cells and uses the enzyme reverse transcriptase?

HIV

What enzyme is deficient in chronic granulomatous disease of childhood?

NADPH oxidase

What rare disorder presents as a large, hard, irregular thyroid gland due to fibrous proliferation of connective tissue in the thyroid gland and extends to adjacent structures?

Riedel thyroiditis

Rheumatic fever most commonly follows pharyngeal infections with what bacteria?

Group A β-hemolytic streptococci

What benign cardiac tumor is associated with tuberous sclerosis?

Rhabdomyoma

What are the rules of 10 regarding pheochromocytoma?

10% are bilateral, 10% malignant, and 10% familial, 10% in children, and 10% outside the adrenal gland

What vascular pathology is associated with HTN in the upper extremities, hypotension in the lower extremities, and a radial-femoral delay?

Postductal coarctation of the aorta (adult)

What seronegative spondyloarthropathy is seen in HLA-B27–positive young females and presents with the triad of conjunctivitis, urethritis, and arthritis affecting the knees and ankles?

Reiter syndrome

What AD disease involves hyperkeratosis of the palms and soles in association with esophageal carcinoma?

Tylosis

A 20-year-old woman who was recently diagnosed with a sexually transmitted disease goes to the ER with a tender, painful, swollen, and erythematous knee (monoarticular). What organism is the likely culprit?

Neisseria gonorrhea (history of STD in patient with monoarticular infectious arthritis: think gonococcus)

What vasculitis is characterized by systemic vasculitis in *small* to *medium*-size vessels (except the lung); affecting young males; 30% *HB$_s$Ag*-positive; *P-ANCA* and autoantibodies against myeloperoxidase?

Polyarteritis nodosa

What malignant bone tumor is associated with familial retinoblastoma?

Osteosarcoma

What bilateral AR disorder seen in infancy as progressive renal failure has multiple small cysts at right angles to the cortical surface?

Polycystic kidney disease of childhood

In what syndrome does the patient have angiomatosis; renal cell carcinomas; pheochromocytomas; retinal, cerebellar, medulla, or spinal cord hemangioblastomas; and epidermal cysts?

von Hippel-Lindau syndrome

What is the term for hyperextension of the PIP and flexion of the DIP joints in rheumatoid arthritis?

Swan-neck deformities

What is the term for white retinal spots surrounded by hemorrhage? In what condition are they seen?

Roth spots, and they are seen in bacterial endocarditis.

A 70-year-old man complains of urinary urgency, nocturia, hesitancy, postvoid dribbling, urinary retention, and a PSA result of 6.5 ng/mL. What is your diagnosis?

BPH. Although an argument can be made for prostatic cancer (you should expect a much higher PSA result), these are buzzwords for BPH. Prostatic cancer is usually silent until late in the disease, when obstructive symptoms begin to occur.

What triad consists of endothelial injury, changes in laminar flow, and hypercoagulation?

Virchow triad, associated with the formation of a thrombus.

What bone cell has receptors for PTH?

Osteoblasts (Remember, they modulate the function of osteoclasts.)

What type of PUD is characterized by the onset of burning epigastric pain immediately after eating?

Gastric ulcer

What is the term for *normal* cellular genes associated with growth and differentiation?

Proto-oncogenes

Blue sclera is seen in what hereditary bone disorder?

Osteogenesis imperfecta

What form of anemia is diagnosed with sucrose lysis test and Ham test?

Paroxysmal nocturnal hemoglobinuria

In what rare AR disorder do you see neutropenia, defective degranulation, and delayed microbial killing due to a problem in chemotaxis and migration?

Chédiak-Higashi syndrome

What myeloid disorder is characterized by increased hematocrit, blood viscosity, basophils, and eosinophils; intense pruritus; and gastric ulcers due to histamine release from basophils, increased LAP, and plethora?

Polycythemia vera (Remember, polycythemia vera is a risk factor for acute leukemias.)

If you order a V/Q scan for suspected pulmonary emboli, is the filling defect seen on the ventilation or perfusion side?

Ventilation of an unperfused lung segment is highly suspicious for pulmonary embolism.

What transports iron in the blood?

Transferrin

What hematological malignancy is particularly likely to affect patients with Down syndrome?

ALL (nearly 15–20 times the normal risk)

What childhood pathology involves anterior bowing of the tibia, epiphyseal enlargements, and costochondral widening, with the endochondral bones being affected?

Rickets

A Japanese man has weight loss, anorexia, early satiety, epigastric abdominal pain, and a palpable left supraclavicular lymph node. On endoscopy you find a large, irregular ulcer with elevated margins on the lesser curvature of the stomach. What is your diagnosis?

Gastric carcinoma

What drug causes a sixfold increase in schizophrenia, can impair motor activity, and can cause lung problems?	Marijuana
What is the term for neurologic signs consistent with a cerebrovascular accident but lasting 24 hours with full recovery?	TIA
What is the name of the tumor when gastric carcinoma spreads to the ovaries?	Krukenberg tumor
What condition results from a deficiency in the enzyme *hexosaminidase A*?	Tay-Sachs disease
Which cerebral herniation results in compression of the anterior cerebral artery?	Cingulate gyrus herniation (subfalcine)
What pathology involves excessive fibrosis throughout the body via increased fibroblast activity, occurs in women more than men, and is most commonly seen in the third to the fifth decade?	Scleroderma
What is the term for the syndrome consisting of hepatomegaly, ascites, and abdominal pain due to hepatic vein thrombosis?	Budd-Chiari syndrome

What form of angina is characterized by

Coronary artery vasospasm, symptom occurrence at rest, ST segment elevation (during episode), and no signs on ECG?	Prinzmetal variant angina
Coronary artery luminal narrowing, symptom occurrence during exertion, ST segment depression on ECG?	Stable angina
Coronary artery nonocclusive thrombus; symptom occurrence with increasing frequency, duration, intensity, and decreasing activity, frequently at rest?	Unstable (crescendo) angina

What skin condition is a localized proliferation of melanocytes presenting as small, oval, light brown macules?	Benign lentigo
What is the term for *nonneoplastic abnormal* proliferation of cell size, shape, and cellular organization?	Dysplasia
What diagnosis ensues from finding well-demarcated erythematous plaques with silvery scales on the knees, elbows, and	Psoriasis

scalp along with nail bed pitting and discoloration?

What renal disease in diabetic patients is seen as a halo of capillaries around the mesangial nodules?	Kimmelstiel-Wilson disease
What autoimmune liver disease is characterized by affecting a middle-aged woman with jaundice, pruritus, fatigue, xanthomas, increased direct bilirubin levels, and *antimitochondrial Abs*?	Primary biliary cirrhosis
What cell in chronic inflammation is derived from blood monocytes?	Macrophages
True or false? Pancreatic insufficiency results in vitamin B_{12} malabsorption.	True. Pancreatic enzymes begin the breakdown of vitamin B_{12}-R complex in the duodenum.
What neuroendocrine tumor produces excess *serotonin*; is associated with diarrhea, flushing, bronchospasms, wheezing; and is diagnosed by findings of elevated *urinary 5-HIAA* levels?	Carcinoid tumor
What tumor constitutes 40% of testicular tumors in children?	Teratoma
What urinary metabolite is elevated in pheochromocytoma?	Vanillylmandelic acid (VMA)

A 25-year-old black woman presents with nonproductive cough, shortness of breath, fatigue, and malaise; she has bilateral hilar lymphadenopathy on chest radiography and elevated ACE levels. What do you diagnose?

Sarcoidosis

What are the four reasons for hypochromic microcytic anemia with a low MCV?

1. Sideroblastic anemias (i.e., porphyrin and heme synthesis disorders)
2. Thalassemia
3. Iron deficiency
4. Lead poisoning

What is characterized by an intense inflammatory reaction, an increase in the amounts of granulation tissue and wound contraction by myofibroblasts?

Healing by secondary intention

What thyroiditis presents as a tender, enlarged, firm thyroid gland, usually preceded by an upper respiratory viral illness?

de Quervain thyroiditis

What disorder leads to IgG autoantibodies to the TSH receptor?

Graves disease

What intrauterine deficiency leads to failure to thrive, mental retardation, motor incoordination, and stunted growth?

Iodine, resulting in congenital hypothyroidism

What pancreatic islet cell tumor is associated with MEN I syndrome?

Gastrinoma

What type of PUD is classically described by the onset of burning epigastric pain 1 to 3 hours after eating that is relieved by food?

Duodenal ulcer

What disease arises from the adrenal medulla, displaces and crosses the midline, metastasizes early, is the most common solid tumor, and is seen in the 2- to 4-year-old age group?

Neuroblastoma

What AD disease associated with chromosome 19 involves a defect in the LDL receptors that leads to skin and tendon xanthomas?

Familial hypercholesterolemia

A 20-year-old woman goes to the ER with ptosis, diplopia, weakness in her jaw muscles when chewing, and muscle *weakness with repeated use*. What is your diagnosis?

Myasthenia gravis

What is the term for RBCs with smooth undulations on the surface of their membrane, commonly seen in uremia?

Burr cells (echinocytes)

Name the cancer associated with the following tumor markers. (Some may have more than one answer.)

β-hCG

Choriocarcinomas and trophoblastic tumors

CA-125	Ovarian cancer
CA-19.9 and CEA	Pancreatic cancer
α-Fetoprotein	Hepatoma and nonseminomatous testicular germ cell tumors
Calcitonin	Medullary carcinoma of the thyroid
PSA and prostatic acid phosphatase	Prostate cancer
Placental alkaline phosphatase	Seminoma
CEA	Cancer of the lung, stomach, colon, and breast

What seronegative spondyloarthropathy is seen in HLA-B27–positive young men, involves the sacroiliac joints, has no subcutaneous nodules, and has a bamboo spine appearance on radiograph?

Ankylosing spondylitis

What disorder is associated with decreased platelet count, prolonged PT and PTT, decreased fibrinogen, and increased fibrin split products (D-dimers)?

Disseminated intravascular coagulation (DIC)

What spirochete is responsible for Lyme disease?

Borrelia burgdorferi

What very aggressive lung cancer metastasizes early and is associated with smoking and paraneoplastic syndromes?

Small cell carcinoma (oat cell)

What bone disorder is characterized by *brown tumors*, bone pain, deformities, and fractures due to *excessive PTH*?	Osteitis fibrosa cystica (von Recklinghausen disease)

What glycogen storage disease is due to the following enzyme deficiencies?

Lysosomal glucosidase (acid maltase)	Pompe's disease
Muscle phosphorylase	McArdle's syndrome
Glucose-6-phosphatase	von Gierke's disease
What ovarian disease involves psammoma bodies?	Serocystadenocarcinoma
What cystic swelling of the chorionic villi is the most common precursor of choriocarcinoma?	Hydatidiform mole
In what condition do you see dimpling on the kidney's surface?	Pyelonephritis

What are the most common causes of osteomyelitis

Overall?	*Staphylococcus aureus*
In neonates?	*Streptococcus agalactiae*
In patients with sickle cell disease?	*Staphylococcus aureus* (but they are more prone to salmonella infections)
In drug addicts?	*Pseudomonas*

What malignant neoplasm of the bone is associated with Homer-Wright pseudorosettes; onion skinning of the periosteum on radiographs of the femur, pelvis, and tibia; and chromosome 11;22 translocation?

Ewing's sarcoma

What lymphoma is characterized by CD19, CD20, CD5; CD23-negative; and chromosome 11;14 translocations?

Mantle cell lymphoma

What components of the complement cascade form the MAC?

C5b–C9

True or false? HPV infection increases the risk of developing squamous cell carcinoma of the penis.

True. HPV serotypes 16 and 18 are risk factors for squamous cell carcinoma.

What form of coarctation of the aorta is associated with Turner syndrome?

Preductal (infantile)

True or false? An elevated serum osteocalcin level is a marker for increased bone formation.

True. Increased alkaline phosphatase levels also are associated with increased bone formation.

What is the most common opportunistic infection of the CNS in HIV?

Toxoplasmosis

What hereditary bone disorder is due to decreased osteoclast function, resulting in thick, sclerotic bones that fracture easily?

Osteopetrosis (Albers-Schönberg disease)

True or false? Pancreatic δ-cell tumors inhibit CCK secretion, leading to gallstones and steatorrhea.

True. δ-Cell tumors produce excess somatostatin, which inhibits CCK, gastrin (hypochlorhydria), and insulin secretion (diabetes).

What is the term for the speckled appearance of the iris in patients with Down syndrome?

Brushfield spots

What is the term for the collapse of the vertebral body due to TB?

Pott disease

What organ must metastasize for carcinoid heart disease to occur?

Liver

Which subset of MEN syndrome is associated with the following?

Medullary carcinoma of the thyroid, pheochromocytoma, and mucocutaneous neuromas

MEN III (or IIb)

Medullary carcinoma of the thyroid, pheochromocytoma, and parathyroid adenomas (or hyperplasia)

MEN IIa (or Sipple syndrome)

Parathyroid, pancreatic, and pituitary gland tumors and Zollinger-Ellison syndrome

MEN I (or Wermer syndrome)

What X-linked recessive disease involves mental retardation, self-mutilation, choreoathetosis, spasticity, a decrease in HGPRT, and an increase in uricemia?

Lesch-Nyhan syndrome

What disorder is associated with spider angiomas, palmar erythema, gynecomastia, testicular atrophy, encephalopathy, abnormalities in clotting factors, and portal HTN?	Cirrhosis
What is your diagnosis of a young, thin asymptomatic female with a midsystolic click on cardiac auscultation?	Mitral valve prolapse
What infection is associated with ring-enhancing lesions seen on computed tomography (CT) of the brain in an HIV-positive individual?	Toxoplasmosis (although you should rule out cerebral abscess due to other organisms)
What is the term for a *reversible* change in one cell type to another?	Metaplasia (usually to a more protective cell type)
What liver tumor is associated with OCP use?	Hepatic adenomas
What CNS developmental abnormality is associated with downward displacement of the cerebellar vermis and medulla compressing the fourth ventricle and leading to obstructive hydrocephalus?	Arnold-Chiari malformation type 2
What disease involves a lack of both T cell-mediated and humoral immune responses that can be either X-linked or AR?	SCID

What condition results in the following CSF results?

Opening pressure 70 to 180 mm H_2O; 0–10 WBCs (monocytes); glucose 45 to 85, protein 15 to 45

Normal values

Opening pressure 450 mm H_2O; 5 WBCs (90% lymphocytes); normal glucose and protein levels

Brain abscess

Opening pressure 100 mm H_2O; 120 WBCs (90% lymphocytes); normal glucose levels; protein 17

Viral meningitis

Opening pressure 250 mm H_2O; WBCs 250 (90% lymphocytes); glucose 35; protein 100

TB meningitis

Opening pressure 400 mm H_2O; WBCs 8500 (90% PMNs); glucose 15; protein 120

Bacterial meningitis

True or false? Removal of the ileum results in vitamin B_{12} deficiencies.

True. The ileum is the site where vitamin B_{12} is absorbed.

What is the term for edema that has LDH below 200, protein level 2.5, and a specific gravity below 1.020?

Transudative; exudative has the opposite values and has an elevated cellular content.

What is the term for thickened, hyperpigmented skin in the axillae, groin, and skin folds associated with malignancies, obesity, and DM?

Acanthosis nigricans

How many grams of protein must be excreted in 24 hours to produce the diagnosis of nephrotic syndrome?

≥ 3.5 g/day of protein, along with generalized edema, hypoalbuminemia, and hyperlipidemia

What illicit drug can cause amyloidosis and focal segmental glomerulosclerosis in the kidney?

Heroin

What catecholamine-hypersecreting tumor, a secondary cause of HTN, results in headache, diaphoresis, anxiety, tachycardia, and palpitations?

Pheochromocytoma

What is the term for flattened nose, low-set ears, and recessed chin seen in patients with bilateral renal agenesis?

Potter facies

What type of healing occurs in a clean surgical incision?

Primary intention

What are the two most common viral infections in HIV?

CMV retinitis and HSV-2

What disorder is defined by inability of the lower esophageal sphincter to relax with swallowing and a bird beak barium swallow result?

Achalasia. (Think Chagas disease if it presents in a person from Central or South America.)

Does Cushing syndrome or Cushing disease have elevated ACTH levels and cortisol suppression with dexamethasone?

Cushing's **disease** (pituitary) has **elevated ACTH** and **cortisol suppression** with dexamethasone, whereas Cushing's **syndrome** (adrenal adenoma) has **decreased ACTH** and **no cortisol suppression** with dexamethasone.

What CD4 T-cell receptor does the HIV virus bind to?

gp120

What is the term for RBC fragments?

Schistocytes

What disorder is due to a deficiency in *tyrosinase*?

Albinism

What two Abs are used to diagnose Hashimoto's thyroiditis?

Antithyroglobulin and antimicrosomal Abs

What urease-producing gram-negative curved rod is associated with PUD and chronic gastritis?

Helicobacter pylori, which is also associated with an increased risk of gastric carcinoma

Name the cancer associated with the following chemical agents. (Some may have more than one answer.)

   Alkylating agents

Leukemias and lymphomas

   Aromatic amines and azo dyes

Hepatocellular carcinoma

Arsenic	Squamous cell carcinoma (skin, lung) and angiosarcoma of the liver
Asbestos	Mesothelioma and bronchogenic carcinoma
Naphthylamine	Bladder cancer
Benzenes	Leukemias
Vinyl chloride	Angiosarcoma of the liver
Chromium and nickel	Bronchogenic carcinoma
Polycyclic aromatic hydrocarbons	Bronchogenic carcinoma
Nitrosamines	Gastric cancer

What are the five conditions associated with normochromic normocytic anemia with a normal MCV and an elevated reticulocyte count?

1. Autoimmune hypersplenism
2. Trauma
3. Anemia
4. Spherocytosis
5. Sickle cell anemia

What pancreatic islet cell tumor is associated with hypoglycemia, sweating, hunger, confusion, and increased C-peptide levels?

Insulinoma

What substance is used to test platelets' response in patients with von Willebrand disease?

Ristocetin

What X-*linked recessive* disorder that is due to an abnormality in dystrophin gene has onset by age 5 with progressive proximal muscle weakness, calf pseudohypertrophy, and elevated CPK levels?

Duchenne muscular dystrophy (Remember, Becker's is slower in progress, less severe, later in onset, and lacks cardiac involvement.)

What subset of adenocarcinoma arises from the terminal bronchioles and/or alveolar walls?	Bronchioloalveolar carcinoma
What estrogen-producing tumor of the female genital tract is characterized by Call-Exner bodies?	Granulosa cell tumor of the ovary
What AD syndrome involves 1000 or more edematous polyps, most commonly affects the colorectal area, and is associated with chromosome 5q21?	Familial polyposis coli
What is the term for osteophyte formation at the *PIP joints* in osteoarthritis? In the *DIP joints?*	Bouchard nodes in the PIP joints; Heberden nodes in the DIP joints.
What prostaglandin is associated with maintaining *patency* of the ductus arteriosus?	PGE (along with low oxygen tension)
What is the term for dilated veins within the spermatic cord?	Varicocele
What type of hemostasis in an intravascular space consists of fibrin, platelets, RBCs, and WBCs?	Thrombus
What is the most common primary malignant tumor in bone?	Osteosarcoma
What is the most common infectious agent in HIV?	*Pneumocystis carinii*

What myeloid disorder is characterized by dry bone marrow aspirations, splenomegaly, leukoerythroblastosis, teardrop RBCs, and hyperuricemia due to increased cell turnover?

Myelofibrosis with myeloid metaplasia

What disease that involves mental retardation, flat face, muscle hypotonia, and a double-bubble sign on radiograph poses an increased risk of Alzheimer's disease and ALL?

Down syndrome (trisomy 21)

What form of anemia is associated with IgG Abs against Rh antigens, positive direct Coombs test, and splenomegaly?

Autoimmune hemolytic anemia

What urinary metabolite is increased in patients with carcinoid syndrome?

5-hydroxyindoleacetic acid (5-HIAA)

What chronic liver disease has a beaded appearance of the bile ducts on cholangiogram?

Primary sclerosing cholangitis

What three LTs are associated with bronchospasms and an increase in vessel permeability and vasoconstriction?

LC_4, LD_4, and LE_4

What are the three Bs of adult polycystic kidneys?

1. **B**ig
2. **B**ilateral
3. **B**erry aneurysm

What AR disease involves a defect in AA 508 on chromosome 7, causing a defect in Cl⁻ transportation that leads to recurrent pulmonary infections and an increase in viscid mucoid secretions along with pancreatic insufficiencies?

Cystic fibrosis. (Parents are usually the first to find out because the baby tastes salty.)

What law states that an enlarged, palpable gallbladder is more likely due to cancer than stone obstruction?

Courvoisier's law

What is the term for air in the pleural space?

Pneumothorax

What disorder of bone remodeling results in thick, weak bones and is associated with high-output cardiac failure?

Paget disease (osteitis deformans)

What is the term to describe the increase in organ size due to the increase in *cell size* and *function*?

Hypertrophy

What slow-growing primary CNS tumor that affects mostly females is associated with psammoma bodies?

Meningioma

True or false? Ethyl alcohol induces the cytochrome P-450 enzymes.

True

What are the five components of portal HTN?

1. Caput medusae
2. Esophageal varices
3. Ascites
4. Splenomegaly
5. Hemorrhoids

What syndrome results when there is a deletion to *paternal* chromosome 15? *Maternal*?

Prader-Willi syndrome and Angelman syndrome, respectively

What CNS tumor arises from Rathke's pouch?

Craniopharyngioma

What is the triad of Reiter syndrome?

1. Peripheral arthritis
2. Conjunctivitis
3. Nongonococcal urethritis

Which of the following is *not* a risk factor for *cholesterol gallstones:* pregnancy, OCP use, female gender, hemolytic anemia, cirrhosis, and obesity? (May be more than one answer.)

Cirrhosis and hemolytic anemia, which are risk factors for **pigmented gallstones.**

Name the nephritic disease based on the immunofluorescent staining.

Mesangial deposits of IgA and C3

IgA nephropathy (Berger disease)

Smooth and linear pattern of IgG and C3 in the GBM

Goodpasture disease

Granular deposits of IgG, IgM, and C3 throughout the glomerulus

Postinfectious GN

What glycoprotein allows platelets to adhere to each other through the use of fibrinogen?

GP IIb/IIIa, which is why GP IIb/IIIa inhibitors are used in the treatment of acute coronary syndromes

What virus is associated with body cavity large B-cell lymphomas?

HHV-8

What germ cell tumor is seen in the 15- to 35-year-old age group, peaks when the person is 35 years of age, and is a bulky mass that spreads via the lymphatic system?

Seminoma

What transmural inflammatory bowel disease can be found from the mouth to anus, has noncaseating granulomas, is discontinuous (skip lesions), and has a cobblestone appearance, thickening of the bowel wall, linear fissures, and aphthous ulcers with normal mucosa between?

Crohn disease

Does ELISA or Western blot confirm whether a patient is HIV-positive?

ELISA screens and **Western blot** confirms the diagnosis.

What GN is highly associated with hepatitis B and C infections?

Membranoproliferative glomerulonephritis (MPGN)

What is the term for squamous to columnar metaplasia of the distal esophagus secondary to chronic inflammation?

Barrett esophagus has an increased risk of developing adenocarcinoma of the esophagus.

What is the term for excessive amounts of granulation tissue that can block re-epithelialization and wound healing?

Proud flesh

What is released from the mitochondria to trigger apoptosis?

Cytochrome c

How much of a vessel must be stenosed to cause sudden cardiac death?	More than 75% of the vessel
Oxidation of Hgb forms what bodies in patients with G-6-PD deficiency?	Heinz bodies
What syndrome that is due to an adrenal gland adenoma produces excess aldosterone resulting in HTN, hypokalemia, and low rennin levels?	Conn syndrome (primary hyperaldosteronism)
What virus is associated with both nasopharyngeal carcinoma and Burkitt lymphoma?	EBV
What normochromic, normocytic AD anemia has splenomegaly and increased osmotic fragility?	Hereditary spherocytosis
What does prepubertal hypersecretion of growth hormone lead to?	Gigantism
What enzyme is deficient in alkaptonuria?	Homogentisic oxidase
What sex cell tumor causes precocious puberty, masculinization, gynecomastia in adults, and crystalloids of Reinke?	Leydig cell tumor
Name four *major* risk factors for atherosclerosis.	DM, hypercholesterolemia, smoking, and HTN are **major** risk factors. Being male, obesity, sedentary lifestyle, homocysteine elevation, OCPs, and genetics are **minor** risk factors for atherosclerosis.

Name the AD disease associated with chromosome 15 in which the patient has long extremities, lax joints, pigeon chest, and posterior mitral leaflet prolapse and is prone to developing dissecting aortic aneurysm.

Marfan syndrome

What is the term for a large VSD that leads to pulmonary HTN, RVH, and cyanosis due to *right-to-left* reversal of the shunt?

Eisenmenger syndrome, which can also occur with any left-to-right shunt

Eating fava beans can produce the Mediterranean type of what deficiency?

G-6-PD deficiency

What form of hemophilia is *X-linked recessive* and due to a deficiency in *factor VIII*?

Hemophilia A

What leukemia affects a 4-year-old child with 3 months of fever, fatigue, generalized lymphadenopathy, CNS involvement, hepatosplenomegaly, bleeding, and platelet count below 100,000?

ALL

What protein deficiency results in respiratory distress syndrome of newborns?

Deficiency in surfactant

What are the three components of amyloid?

1. Fibrillary protein
2. Amyloid protein
3. Glycosaminoglycans

What autoimmune disorder is due to Abs directed to ACh receptors at the NMJ?	Myasthenia gravis
What are the three left-to-right shunts?	1. VSD 2. ASD 3. PDA
What protein causes fibrinolysis?	Plasmin
What pancreatic islet cell tumor is associated with watery diarrhea, hypokalemia, and achlorhydria?	VIPoma
True or false? Obesity, DM, HTN, multiparity, early menarche, and late menopause are all risk factors for endometrial carcinoma.	False. They are all risk factors for endometrial carcinoma except multiparity. Nulliparity, estrogen-producing tumors, and estrogen replacement therapy are also risk factors for endometrial carcinoma.
What is the term for pigmented iris hamartomas seen in patients with neurofibromatosis type 1?	Lisch nodules
What GI pathology is associated with a positive string sign, an increase in the number of bloody stools, RLQ pain, skip lesions, terminal ileum most commonly affected, occurrence in women more than men, and an increased thickness of the bowel?	Crohn disease
What is the most common fungal infection in HIV?	*Candida*

True or false? GERD is a cause of asthma.

True. Don't forget this in your differential diagnosis of an asthmatic.

Name the product or products of *arachidonic acid*:

Vasodilation and inhibition of platelet aggregation produced by vascular endothelium

PGI_2

Vasodilation

PGE_2, PGD_2, and PGF_2

Pain and fever

PGE_2

Vasoconstriction and platelet aggregation produced by platelets

TXA_2

Chemotactic for neutrophils

LTB_4

Vasodilation, bronchospasm, and increased vascular permeability

LTC_4, LTD_4, and LTE_4

Which hepatitis B *Ab* indicates low transmissibility?

HB_eAb

What pneumoconiosis is associated with exposure to the following *occupations* or *materials*?

Miners, metal grinders, and sandblasters

Silicosis

***Aerospace* industry, nuclear reactors**

Berylliosis

Shipyards, brake linings, *insulation*, and old building construction	Asbestosis Note: Coal worker's pneumoconiosis is synonymous with black lung disease, an upper lobe occupational disorder
What is the term for calcification of the gallbladder seen on radiograph due to chronic cholecystitis or adenocarcinoma of the gallbladder?	Porcelain gallbladder
What is the term to describe a decrease in the cell size and function usually associated with disuse?	**Atrophy.** Disuse can also be due to immobilization, ischemia, aging, and a host of other causes.
Which B-cell neoplasm has the following cell surface markers: CD19, CD20, CD5 (T-cell marker), CD23; and are CD10-negative?	CLL (B-cell origin)
What disease caused by decompression sickness leads to multiple foci of ischemic necrosis that affect the head of the femur, humerus, and tibia?	Caisson disease
What are the four DNA oncogenic viruses?	1. HPV 2. EBV 3. Hepatitis B 4. Kaposi sarcoma
Is the AD or AR form of osteopetrosis malignant?	The **AR** form is malignant and AD is benign.
What carcinoma produces hematuria, flank pain, and a palpable mass?	This is the triad of renal cell carcinoma

Name at least three causes of metastatic calcification.	Remember the mnemonic **PAM SMIDT** **P,** (hyper)**P**arathyroid/**P**aget disease **A,** Addison's disease **M,** Milk-alkali syndrome/metastatic cancer **S,** Sarcoidosis **M,** Multiple myeloma **I,** Immobilization/idiopathic **D,** Vitamin D intoxication **T,** Tumors
What is the only subtype of Hodgkin's lymphoma that is most commonly seen in females?	Nodular sclerosis
What is the leading cause of preventable premature death and illness in the United States?	Smoking
What prion-associated CNS pathology produces rapidly progressive dementia with myoclonus, involuntary movements, and death within 6 to 12 months?	Creutzfeldt-Jakob disease
What breast malignancy has tumor cells with a halo surrounding the nucleus and is an ulceration of the nipple and areola with crusting, fissuring, and oozing?	Paget disease of the breast
What breast pathology involves malignant cells with halos invading the epidermis of the skin?	Paget disease of the breast
Macro-ovalocytes in the peripheral blood smear are formed from what cell in the bone marrow?	Megaloblasts

Name the type of *exudate*, given the following examples.

Sunburn	Serous exudates
Uremic pericarditis	Fibrinous exudates
Parasitic infection	Eosinophilic exudates
***Diphtheria* infection**	Pseudomembranous exudates
Meningococcal infection	Purulent exudates
Rickettsial infection	Hemorrhagic exudates

What parasite is associated with squamous cell carcinoma of the urinary bladder?

Schistosoma haematobium

What malabsorption syndrome produces abdominal distention, bloating, flatulence, diarrhea, steatorrhea, and weight loss shortly after eating bread products?

Celiac sprue (gluten-sensitive enteropathy)

What herpes virus is associated with Kaposi sarcoma?

HHV 8

What is the term for the copper corneal deposits found in Wilson's disease?

Kayser-Fleischer rings

Name the six vitamin K–dependent coagulation factors.

Factors II, VII, IX, and X and proteins C and S.

What ovarian carcinoma is characterized by psammoma bodies?

Cystadenocarcinoma

A *marfanoid* patient presents with *tearing* retrosternal chest pain *radiating to her back*. What is your first diagnosis?	Dissecting aortic aneurysm. MI is also high on the list, but the highlighted words are buzzwords to look for dissection.
What malignant neoplasm of the skin is associated with keratin pearls?	Squamous cell carcinoma
Name four chemotactic factors for neutrophils.	N-formyl-methionine, LTB4, C5a, and IL-8
What is the term for granuloma at the lung apex in TB?	Simon focus
What are the three platelet aggregating factors?	1. ADP 2. PG 3. TXA_2
What syndrome is due to a *Neisseria* sp. infection in a child resulting in bilateral hemorrhagic infarcts of the adrenal glands?	Waterhouse-Friderichsen syndrome
What foci of fibrinoid necrosis are surrounded by lymphocytes and macrophages throughout all the layers of the heart?	Aschoff bodies of rheumatic fever
What is the leading cause of primary hyperparathyroidism?	Chief cell adenoma (80%)
In what X-linked recessive disease is there a decrease in the HMP shunt, along with Heinz body formation?	G-6-PD deficiency

What is the term for a RBC that has a peripheral rim of Hgb with a dark central Hgb-containing area?

Target cell

True or false? Raynaud's phenomenon has no underlying pathology.

False. The **disease** has no associated pathology; the **phenomenon** is arterial insufficiency due to an underlying disease.

What benign solitary papillary growth within the lactiferous ducts of the breast commonly produces bloody nipple discharge?

Intraductal papilloma

What form of hemophilia is X-*linked recessive* and is due to a deficiency in *factor IX*?

Hemophilia B

What are the two reasons for megaloblastic anemia with elevated MCV?

Vitamin B_{12} deficiency and folate deficiency

Is cigarette smoking associated with transitional cell carcinoma of the bladder?

Yes. It is also a cause of cancers of the lung, esophagus, ureter, and kidney, just to name a few.

What disease has multiple schwannomas, café-au-lait spots on the skin, and Lisch nodules and is associated with chromosome 17q?

Neurofibromatosis I (chromosome 22q is with neurofibromatosis II and no Lisch nodules)

What syndrome is due to Abs directed to calcium channels and causes muscle *weakness that improves with repeated use*?

Eaton-Lambert syndrome

In what rare lung malignancy have 90% of patients had an occupational exposure to *asbestos*?

Malignant mesothelioma

What is the term for cytoplasmic remnants of RNA in RBCs, seen in lead poisoning?

Basophilic stippling

What is the triad of fat embolism?

1. Petechiae
2. Hyperactive mental status
3. Occurrence within 24 to 48 hours of the initial insult (e.g., long bone fracture)

Upon seeing negatively birefringent needle-shaped crystals from a joint aspiration of the great toe, what form of arthritis do you diagnose?

Gout

What condition is manifested by bilateral sarcoidosis of the parotid glands, submaxillary gland, and submandibular gland with posterior uveal tract involvement?

Mikulicz syndrome

What female genital tract disorder is characterized by obesity, hirsutism, infertility, amenorrhea, elevated LH and testosterone levels, and low FSH levels?

Polycystic ovary disease (Stein-Leventhal syndrome)

What bronchogenic carcinoma is associated with an elevated level of Ca^{2+}, involves keratin pearls, occurs in men more than women, is associated with smoking, occurs in the major bronchi, and is seen in the central areas of the lung?

Squamous cell carcinoma

What disorder is due to a deficiency in the enzyme *phenylalanine hydroxylase*?

PKU

True or false? Being a white male increases your risk factor for testicular cancer.

Oddly enough, it is true. Cryptorchidism, Klinefelter syndrome, testicular feminization, and family history of testicular cancer are all risk factors.

Can an acute MI be diagnosed *only* by looking at an ECG?

No. Remember, tests do not diagnose, they confirm or refute your diagnosis. Also, diagnosis of MI requires two of three criteria: chest pain consistent and characteristic of MI, elevated cardiac enzymes consistent with MI, and ST segment elevation of 2 mm or more in at least two contiguous leads.

What autoimmune syndrome is characterized by keratoconjunctivitis, corneal ulcers, xerostomia, and an increased risk of high-grade B-cell lymphomas? What two Ab tests are used in making the diagnosis?

Sjögren's syndrome; SS-A (Ro) and SS-B (La)

True or false? Sickle cell anemia, Caisson disease, chronic steroid use, and Gaucher disease are causes of avascular necrosis of bone.

True. Fractures and trauma, however, are the most common causes.

What gene *stimulates* apoptosis when DNA repair is unable to be done?

p-53

Is ulcerative colitis or Crohn disease *more commonly* associated with primary sclerosing cholangitis?

Ulcerative colitis

What test uses p24 protein when diagnosing HIV?

ELISA test

How many café-au-lait spots are necessary for the diagnosis of neurofibromatosis type 1?

At least six

What is the term for severe and protracted *vomiting* resulting in *linear* lacerations at the gastroesophageal junction?

Mallory-Weiss syndrome

What is the term for hypercalcemia resulting in precipitation of calcium phosphate in *normal tissue*?

Metastatic calcification

What is the term for a twisting of the bowel around its vascular axis resulting in intestinal obstruction?

Volvulus

What form of poisoning is associated with *bitter almond*–scented breath?

Cyanide

Name the type of hypersensitivity reaction based on the following properties.

Circulating *Ab-Ag immune complexes* deposited in the tissue result in neutrophil attraction and the release of lysosomal enzymes.

Type III hypersensitivity (immune complex)

IgE-mediated release of chemical mediators from basophils and mast cells; need prior exposure to Ag in the past; eosinophils amplify and continue reaction; can be system or localized.	Type I hypersensitivity (anaphylactic)
IgG or IgM Abs against a specific target cell or tissue; *complement-dependent* or ADCC.	Type II hypersensitivity (cytotoxic)
Reaction-mediated by sensitized T-cells	Type IV hypersensitivity (cell-mediated)
What highly undifferentiated aggressive CNS tumor of primordial neuroglial origin develops in children and is associated with pseudorosettes?	Primitive neuroectodermal tumors (i.e., medulloblastomas and retinoblastomas)
What syndrome is due to anti-GBM Abs directed against the lung and kidneys?	Goodpasture syndrome
What pathway of the coagulation cascade is activated when it is in contact with *foreign surfaces*?	**Intrinsic.** The extrinsic pathway is activated by the release of tissue factors.
What tumor is seen in the 2- to 4-year-old age group; does not cross the midline; has immature glomeruli, tubules, and stroma; and metastasizes late to the lungs?	Wilms tumor

What CNS tumor commonly produces tinnitus and hearing loss?	Schwannoma
True or false? Anticentromere Abs are used in diagnosing CREST syndrome.	True. Scl-70 Abs are used in diagnosing diffuse scleroderma.
What AR CNS disorder presents early in childhood with gait ataxia, loss of deep tendon reflexes, impaired vibratory sensation, hand clumsiness, and loss of position sense?	Friedreich ataxia
What potent platelet aggregator and vasoconstrictor is synthesized by platelets?	TXA_2
Which type of cerebral herniation is associated with CN III palsy?	Transtentorial (uncal)
What form of vasculitis involves the *ascending* arch and causes *obliterative endarteritis* of the *vasa vasorum*?	Syphilitic
What is the main type of cell involved in cellular immunity?	T lymphocyte
What skin condition has irregular blotchy patches of hyperpigmentation on the face commonly associated with OCP use and pregnancy?	Melasma

What is the classic triad of TB?

Fever, night sweats, and hemoptysis

True or false? Blood clots lack platelets.

True. A thrombus has platelets, but clots do not.

What malignant tumor of the skin is associated with Birbeck granules?

Histiocytosis X

What type of anemia is the result of a deficiency in intrinsic factor?

Pernicious anemia (secondary to a lack of vitamin B_{12} absorption)

What cancer is particularly likely to affect English chimney sweeps?

Scrotal cancer, due to the high exposure to polycyclic aromatic hydrocarbons

What is the term for a raised fluid-filled cavity greater than 0.5 cm that lies between the layers of the skin?

Bulla

What virus is associated with the endemic form of Burkitt lymphoma?

EBV

With which pituitary adenoma is an elevated *somatomedin C* level associated?

GH-producing adenoma

What three criteria allow you to differentiate an ulcer from an erosion or carcinoma?

1. Less than 3 cm
2. Clean base
3. Level with the surrounding mucosa

Name the four right-to-left congenital cardiac shunts.

Truncus arteriosus, **T**ricuspid atresia, **T**ransposition of the great vessels, and **T**etralogy of Fallot. (They all begin with **T.**)

What do low levels of Ca^{2+} and PO_4 along with

Hypoparathyroidism

neuromuscular irritability indicate?

Does PT or PTT test the *extrinsic* coagulation pathway?

PT for extrinsic and PTT for intrinsic (remember: wPeT and hPiTT, which means warfarin, extrinsic, PT; heparin, intrinsic, PTT)

What leukemia is associated with four-leaf-clover lymphocytes on peripheral blood smear?

Adult T-cell leukemia

What ring is a weblike narrowing of the gastroesophageal junction?

Schatzki ring

With what disease do you see IgA deposits in small vessels of the skin and the kidneys?

Henoch-Schönlein purpura

What rapidly progressive and aggressive T-cell lymphoma affects young males with a mediastinal mass (thymic)?

Lymphoblastic lymphoma

What is the term for the appearance of the kidney in malignant hypertension (it has petechiae on its surface)?

Flea-bitten kidney (can also be seen in pyelonephritis)

True or false? Psammoma bodies are seen in *medullary* carcinoma of the thyroid.

False. Elevated calcitonin levels are seen in medullary carcinoma of the thyroid. **Psammoma bodies** are seen in **papillary carcinoma** of the **thyroid** and **ovaries,** as well as **meningiomas.**

What is the lecithin:sphingomyelin ratio in respiratory distress syndrome of newborns?

< 2

What syndrome has loss of deep tendon reflexes, muscle weakness, and ascending paralysis preceded by a viral illness?	Guillain-Barré syndrome
What form of endocarditis do patients with SLE commonly encounter?	Libman-Sacks endocarditis
What is the term for black pigmentation of the colon associated with laxative abuse?	Melanosis coli
Are the following major or minor Jones criteria of rheumatic fever?	
Fever	Minor
Migratory polyarthritis	Major
Subcutaneous nodules	Major
Elevated acute phase reactants (e.g., ESR)	Minor
Arthralgias	Minor
Pericarditis	Major
Erythema marginatum	Major
Sydenham chorea	Major
What gene *inhibits* apoptosis by preventing the release of cytochrome *c* from mitochondria?	*Bcl-2*
Which hepatitis strain is a defective virus that can replicate only inside HBV-infected cells?	Hepatitis D

What are the three main components of amyloid?

Fibrillary protein, amyloid protein, and glycosaminoglycans (heparin sulfate mainly)

What leukemia is characterized by Philadelphia chromosomal translocation (9;22); massive splenomegaly; peripheral leukocytosis (commonly > 100,00); decreased LAP levels; and nonspecific symptoms of fatigue, malaise, weight loss, and anorexia?

CML

What is the difference between a Ghon focus and a Ghon complex?

A Ghon focus is a TB tubercle, whereas a Ghon complex is a focus with hilar lymph node involvement.

In what disease do you see horseshoe kidneys, rockerbottom feet, low-set ears, micrognathia, and mental retardation?

Edward syndrome (trisomy 18)

What parasitic infection is associated with cholangiocarcinoma?

Clonorchis sinensis

What disorder is associated with loss of polarity, anaplasia, pleomorphism, discohesiveness, increase in the nuclear:cytoplasmic ratio, hyperchromasia, and increase in the rate of mitosis?

Malignancy

What is the term for telescoping of the proximal bowel into the distal segment presenting as abdominal pain, *currant jelly* stools, and intestinal obstruction?

Intussusception

What mushroom poisoning is associated with fulminant hepatitis with extensive liver necrosis? — *Amanita phalloides*

What type of erythema do you see in

    Ulcerative colitis? — Erythema nodosum

    Rheumatic fever? — Erythema marginatum

    Stevens-Johnson syndrome? — Erythema multiforme

What benign bone tumor is associated with Gardner syndrome? — Osteoma

What renal calculus is associated with urea-splitting bacteria? — Magnesium ammonium phosphate (struvite)

What lymphoma is associated with bleeding and cryoglobulin precipitation at low temperatures, headache and confusion due to hyperviscosity, IgM M-protein spike on serum electrophoresis, and Russell bodies? — Waldenström's macroglobulinemia

What type of acute metal poisoning involves stomach and colon erosion and acute tubular necrosis? — Mercury

What slow-growing CNS tumor in 30- to 50-year-old — Oligodendroglioma

patients with a long history of seizures has fried egg cellular appearance in a network of chicken wire?

Goodpasture Ag is a component of what type of collagen?

Type IV collagen

If a peripheral blood smear shows *schistocytes*, *reticulocytes*, and *thrombocytopenia*, is it more commonly seen in patients with ITP or TTP?

TTP; thrombocytopenia with megathrombocytes is more characteristic of ITP.

After traveling in a plane across the Atlantic Ocean, an obese male goes to the ER with swollen right leg and sudden onset of shortness of breath. What do you immediately diagnose?

Pulmonary embolism due to a DVT; this is not absolute but a classic description.

What cell type involves humoral immunity?

B lymphocyte

What is the first sign of megaloblastic anemia on a peripheral blood smear?

Hypersegmented neutrophils

What is the term for gastric ulcers associated with severely burned or traumatic patients?

Curling ulcers (think curling iron = burn)

What syndrome arises from mutation in the *fibrillin gene (FBN1)* on chromosome 15q21?

Marfan syndrome

What AD disorder is characterized by degeneration of GABA neurons in the caudate nucleus resulting in atrophy, chorea, dementia, and personality changes?

Huntington disease

What atypical pneumonia can be diagnosed with elevated cold agglutinin titers?

Mycoplasma pneumoniae

What is the triad of Felty syndrome?

Neutropenia, splenomegaly, and rheumatoid arthritis

What is the term for the *unidirectional* attraction of cells toward a chemical mediator released during inflammation?

Chemotaxis

What is the term for a benign melanocytic tumor associated with sun exposure that presents as tan-to-brown colored and has sharply defined well-circumscribed borders?

Benign nevus (mole)

What *small-* to *medium-*sized vasculitis is seen in a 35-year-old *man* who is a *heavy smoker* presenting with claudication symptoms in the upper and lower extremities?

Buerger disease (thromboangiitis obliterans)

What is the term for pelvic inflammatory disease of the fallopian tubes?

Salpingitis

What disease with familial mental retardation produces large, everted ears and macro-orchidism?	Fragile X syndrome
What type of skin carcinoma occurring on sun-exposed sites has a low level of metastasis?	Squamous cell carcinoma
What is the tetrad of tetralogy of Fallot?	VSD, RVH, overriding aorta, and pulmonary stenosis
What is the term for chronic necrotizing pulmonary infections resulting in permanent airway dilation and associated with Kartagener syndrome?	Bronchiectasis
What is an elevated, fluid-filled cavity between skin layers up to 0.5 cm?	Vesicle (e.g., poison ivy)
What is the term for panhypopituitarism secondary to ischemic necrosis and hypotension postpartum?	Sheehan syndrome
What disease is diagnosed by findings of ANAs and anti-SCL-70 antibodies?	Scleroderma
What is the name of the ovarian cyst containing ectodermal, endodermal, and mesodermal elements (i.e., skin, hair, teeth and neural tissue)?	Teratoma (dermoid cyst)

What syndrome is seen in *iron-deficient* middle-aged women with *esophageal webs*?

Plummer-Vinson syndrome

What are the three causes of transudate?

CHF, cirrhosis, and nephrosis

A chronic alcohol abuser goes to the ER with weakness, a sore, beefy red tongue, loss of vibration and position sense, arm and leg dystaxia, elevated levels of methylmalonic acid in the urine, and anemia with an MCV above 105 fL. What is your diagnosis, and how will you monitor his response to treatment?

Subacute combined degeneration of the spinal cord is treated with **IM vitamin B_{12}** injections. If treatment is working, you will see an **increased reticulocyte count** on the peripheral smear in about 5 days.

What form of GN is characteristically associated with crescent formation?

Rapidly progressive glomerulonephritis (RPGN)

What vitamin deficiency may result in sideroblastic anemia?

Vitamin B_6

What is the term for TB with the cervical lymph node involved?

Scrofula

***Influx* of what ion is associated with irreversible cell injury?**

Massive influx of **calcium**

What pathology is associated with elevated levels of Ca^{2+}, cardiac arrhythmias, bone resorption, kidney stones,

Primary hyperparathyroidism

and metastatic calcifications?

What type of metal poisoning causes mental retardation, somnolence, convulsions, and encephalopathy?

Lead

What syndrome is rheumatoid arthritis with pneumoconiosis?

Caplan syndrome

True or false? All of the following are risk factors for cervical cancer: multiple pregnancies, early age of intercourse, multiple sexual partners, OCP use, smoking, HIV, and STDs.

True. Don't forget this list; you will be asked.

What is the term for precipitation of calcium phosphate in *dying* or *necrotic tissue*?

Dystrophic calcification

What congenital small bowel outpouching is a remnant of the vitelline duct?

Meckel diverticulum

What type of crystals are associated with gout?

Monosodium urate crystals

What is the term for transverse bands on the *fingernails* seen in patients with *chronic arsenic* poisoning?

Mees lines

What is the tumor at the bifurcation of the right and left hepatic ducts?

Klatskin tumor

IgE-mediated mast cell release, C3a and C5a, and IL-1 all trigger the release of what vasoactive amine?	Histamine
What disease is seen in the 20- to 40-year-old age group, is more prevalent in women than men, involves diarrhea with or without bloody stools, starts in the rectum and ascends without skipping areas, includes pseudopolyps, and has a thickness of the bowel that does not change?	Ulcerative colitis
What disorder causes joint stiffness that *worsens with repetitive motion*, crepitus, effusions, and swelling and commonly affects the knees, hips, and spine?	Osteoarthritis
What condition is characterized by a 46XY karyotype, testes present, and ambiguous or female external genitalia?	Male pseudohermaphrodite (dude looks like a lady!)
What is the term for RBC remnants of nuclear chromatin in asplenic patients?	Howell-Jolly bodies
What is the term for gastric ulcers associated with increased intracranial pressure?	Cushing's ulcers
What platelet disorder is characteristically seen in *children* following a bout of	Hemolytic uremic syndrome

gastroenteritis with *bloody diarrhea*?

Are elevated alkaline phosphatase and decreased phosphorus and calcium levels more consistent with osteoporosis or osteomalacia?

Osteomalacia. Osteoporosis has normal levels of calcium, phosphorus, and alkaline phosphatase.

What vascular tumor associated with von Hippel-Lindau syndrome involves the cerebellum, brainstem, spinal cord, and retina?

Hemangioblastoma

How many segments in a neutrophilic nucleus are necessary for it to be called *hypersegmented*?

At least 5 lobes

Name the type of regeneration (i.e., labile, stable, or permanent) based on the following examples.

Epidermis	Labile
Skeletal muscle	Permanent
Pancreas	Stable
CNS neurons	Permanent
Fibroblasts	Stable
Hematopoietic cells	Labile
Liver	Stable
Smooth muscle	Stable

Cardiac muscle	Permanent
Mucosal epithelium	Labile
Kidney	Stable
Osteoblasts	Stable (**Labile** cells proliferate throughout life; **stable** cells have a low level of proliferation; and **permanent** cells as the name states, do not proliferate.)

What CNS tumor cells stain positive for glial fibrillary acidic protein (GFAP)?

Astrocytoma

True or false? Elevated ASO titers and serum complement levels are associated with poststreptococcal GN.

False. ASO titers are elevated, but serum complement levels are decreased.

What glycoprotein allows platelets to adhere to von Willebrand factor?

GP Ib

What encephalitis is associated with the *JC virus*?

Progressive multifocal leukoencephalopathy

Hereditary angioneurotic edema (AD) produces local edema in organs (e.g., GI, skin, respiratory tract). What enzyme deficiency causes increased capillary permeability due to a release of vasoactive peptides?

C1 esterase inhibitor (C1INH)

Is an anti-HAV IgG Ab associated with immunization or recent infection?

Anti-HAV IgG Abs are associated with **immunization** or a **prior infection.** **Anti-HAV IgM** is associated with **acute** or **recent infection.**

Which integrin mediates adhesion by binding to lymphocyte function–associated Ag 1 (LFA-1) and MAC-1 leukocyte receptors?

Intercellular adhesion molecule (ICAM) 1

Name the cerebral vessel associated with the following vascular pathologies.

Subarachnoid hemorrhage

Berry aneurysm in the circle of Willis

Subdural hemorrhage

Bridging veins draining into the sagittal sinus

Epidural hemorrhage

Middle meningeal artery

True or false? Live vaccines are contraindicated in patients with SCID.

True

What is the term for the round intracytoplasmic eosinophilic inclusions containing α-synuclein found in the dopaminergic neurons of the substantia nigra?

Lewy bodies

In which form of emphysema, panacinar or centriacinar, is the effect worse in the apical segments of the upper lobes?

Centriacinar worse in upper lobes; panacinar worse in base of lower lobes

What syndrome results if the enzyme α-1-iduronidase is deficient? *L-iduronate sulfatase* **deficiency?**

Hurler syndrome and Hunter syndrome, respectively

What percentage of the bone marrow must be composed of blast for leukemia to be considered?

At least 30% blast in the bone marrow

What is the term for the heart's inability to maintain perfusion and meet the metabolic demands of tissues and organs?

CHF

What syndrome occurs when pelvic inflammatory disease ascends to surround the liver capsule in violin string adhesions?

Fitz-Hugh-Curtis syndrome

True or false? Patients with Turner syndrome have no Barr bodies.

True. Remember, the second X chromosome is inactivated, and so is the Barr body. Turner syndrome has only one X chromosome.

What is the term for the sign revealed when a psoriatic scale is removed and pinpoint bleeding occurs?

Auspitz sign

What type of Hgb is increased in patients with sickle cell anemia who take hydroxyurea?

Hgb F

What vasculitis affects a 30-year-old *Asian female* **having visual field deficits, dizziness, decreased blood pressure, and** *weakened pulses* **in the** *upper extremities*?

Takayasu arteritis (medium-size to large vessels)

A 20-year-old college student has fever, grey-white membranes over the tonsils, posterior auricular lymphadenitis, and hepatosplenomegaly. What is your diagnosis? What test do you order to confirm your diagnosis?

EBV infections resulting in **infectious mononucleosis** can be diagnosed by the **Monospot test.** (Remember, it may be negative in the first week of the illness, so retest if you have a high index of suspicion.)

What cell type is commonly elevated in asthma?

Eosinophil

What pathology is associated with deposition of calcium pyrophosphate in patients older than 50 years?

Pseudogout

What thyroid carcinoma secretes *calcitonin* and arises from the parafollicular C cells?

Medullary carcinoma of the thyroid

What illegal drug can cause rhabdomyolysis, MI, cerebral infarct, and lethal cardiac arrhythmias?

Cocaine

What AA is substituted for glutamic acid at position 6 on the β-chain in patients with sickle cell anemia?

Valine

What endogenous pigment found in the substantia nigra and melanocytes is formed by the *oxidation of tyrosine* to dihydroxyphenylalanine?

Melanin

What tumor marker is associated with seminomas?

Placental alkaline phosphatase

What type of GN, associated with celiac disease and dermatitis herpetiformis, has mesangial deposits of IgA, C3, properdin, IgG, and IgM?	Berger disease (IgA nephropathy)
What AD disease is associated with chromosome 4p; does not present until the person is in his or her 30s; and involves atrophy of the caudate nucleus, dilatation of the lateral and third ventricles, and signs of extrapyramidal lesions?	Huntington disease
What pattern of inheritance is G-6-PD deficiency?	X-linked recessive
What adenocarcinoma presents with elevated levels of acid phosphatase, dihydrotestosterone, PSA, and bone pain?	Prostatic carcinoma
Is Dubin-Johnson or Rotor syndrome associated with black pigmentation of the liver?	Both are **AR** with conjugated hyperbilirubinemia, but **Dubin-Johnson syndrome** is differentiated from Rotor by the black pigmentation of the liver.
What oxygen-dependent killing enzyme requires hydrogen peroxide and halide (Cl^-) to produce hypochlorous acid?	Myeloperoxidase
What condition results in a strawberry gallbladder?	Cholesterolosis
What three chemical agents are associated with angiosarcomas of the liver?	Arsenic, thorotrast, and vinyl chloride

What is the term for programmed cell death?	Apoptosis (Remember, there is a lack of inflammatory response.)
What potentially fatal disease occurs in children who are given ASA during a viral illness?	Reye syndrome
What metal poisoning produces microcytic anemia with *basophilic stippling*?	Lead poisoning
What inflammatory bowel disorder is continuous, with extensive ulcerations and pseudopolyps, and is associated with HLA-B27?	Ulcerative colitis
What is the pentad of TTP?	Neurologic symptoms Renal failure Thrombocytopenia Fever Microangiopathic hemolytic anemia (Don't forget it. When I was an intern, my senior resident asked me this question more times than I would like to remember.)
Which hepatitis B *Ag* correlates with infectivity and viral proliferation?	HB_eAg
What disease involves cold skin abscesses due to a defect in neutrophil chemotaxis and a serum IgE level higher than 2000?	Job syndrome
What female pathology is associated with endometrial glands and stroma outside the uterus commonly affecting the ovaries as chocolate cysts?	Endometriosis

What is the karyotype in Turner syndrome?	45XO
What is the term for a congenital absence of the ganglionic cells of the Auerbach and Meissner plexus in the rectum and sigmoid colon?	Hirschsprung disease (aganglionic megacolon)
What syndrome is associated with gastrin-producing islet cell tumor resulting in multiple intractable peptic ulcers?	Zollinger-Ellison syndrome
What type of collagen is associated with keloid formation?	Type III
The "tea-and-toast" diet is classically associated with what cause of megaloblastic anemia?	Folate deficiency (very common in the elderly)
What is the term for ascending bacterial infection of the renal pelvis, tubules, and interstitium causing costovertebral angle tenderness, fever, chills, dysuria, frequency, and urgency?	Pyelonephritis
How can a deficiency in adenosine deaminase be a bone marrow suppressor?	It causes a buildup of dATP, which inhibits ribonucleotide reductase and leads to a decrease in deoxynucleoside triphosphate, a precursor of DNA, resulting in overall bone marrow suppression.
Which phenotype of osteogenesis imperfecta is incompatible with life?	Type II

With what is cherry red intoxication associated?	Acute CO poisoning
What are the four most common causes of femoral head necrosis?	1. Steroids 2. Alcohol 3. Scuba diving 4. Sickle cell anemia
What are the four signs of acute inflammation?	Rubor (red), dolor (pain), calor (heat), tumor (swelling); also sometimes there is loss of function

Name the hypochromic microcytic anemia based on the following laboratory values.

Increased iron, decreased TIBC, increased percent saturation, increased ferritin	Sideroblastic anemia
Decreased iron, TIBC, and percent saturation; increased ferritin	Anemia of chronic disease
Decreased iron, percent saturation, and ferritin; increased TIBC	Iron deficiency anemia
Normal iron, TIBC, percent saturation, and ferritin	Thalassemia minor
Which form of emphysema is associated with an α_1-antitrypsin deficiency?	Panacinar
An 80-year-old woman presents to you with right-sided temporal headache, facial pain and blurred vision on the affected side, and an elevated ESR. Your diagnosis?	Temporal arteritis (giant cell arteritis)

What type of neurofibromatosis is associated with bilateral acoustic schwannomas?

Type 2

What disorder is due to a deficiency in the enzyme *glucocerebrosidase*?

Gaucher disease

What is the term for flexion of the PIP and extension of the DIP joints seen in rheumatoid arthritis?

Boutonnière deformities

True or false? Atelectasis is an *irreversible* collapse of a lung.

False. Atelectasis is a **reversible** collapse of a lung.

What viral infection in patients with sickle cell anemia results in aplastic crisis?

Parvovirus B 19

What syndrome has elevated FSH and LH levels with decreased testosterone levels and 47XXY karyotype?

Klinefelter syndrome

What CNS developmental abnormality is associated with 90% of syringomyelia?

Arnold-Chiari malformation type 2

What is the term for fibrinoid necrosis of the arterioles in the kidney secondary to malignant hypertension?

Onion skinning

A 30-year-old woman goes to your office with bilateral multiple breast nodules that vary with menstruation

Fibrocystic change of the breast. This highlights the distinguishing features from breast cancer, which is commonly unilateral, single nodule, no variation with

and have cyclical pain and engorgement. What is your diagnosis?

menstruation, and no changes during pregnancy.

What disease is X-linked recessive, is associated with eczema thrombocytopenia and an increased chance of developing recurrent infections, involves a decrease in serum IgM and in the T cell-dependent paracortical areas of the lymph nodes, and means that the patient is likely to develop malignant lymphoma?

Wiskott-Aldrich syndrome

Which form of melanoma carries the worst prognosis?

Nodular melanoma

Patients with sickle cell anemia are at increased risk for infection from what type of organisms?

Encapsulated bacteria

How many major and/or minor Jones criteria are required for the diagnosis of rheumatic fever?

Two major or one major and two minor

What skin carcinoma is a superficial dermal infiltrate of T lymphocytes seen in males more than 40 years old and presents as scaly red patches or plaques?

Mycosis fungoides (cutaneous T-cell lymphoma)

What *Hgb*-derived endogenous pigment is found in areas of hemorrhage or bruises?

Hemosiderin

What is a palpable, elevated solid mass up to 0.5 cm?	Papule
True or false? Monocytosis is seen in TB.	True
What pathology is associated with podagra, tophi in the ear, and PMNs with monosodium urate crystals?	Gout
What GI pathology can be caused by a patient taking clindamycin or lincomycin or by *Clostridium difficile*, ischemia, *Staphylococcus*, *Shigella*, or *Candida* infection?	Pseudomembranous colitis
What do the risk factors late menopause, early menarche, obesity, nulliparity, excessive estrogen, genetic factor p53, and *brc-abl* characterize?	Breast cancer
What thyroid carcinoma is associated with radiation exposure, psammoma bodies, and Orphan Annie eye nuclei?	Papillary carcinoma of the thyroid
Name three opsonins.	Fc portion of IgG, C3b, and mannose-binding proteins
What chemical can be dangerous if you work in the aerospace industry or in nuclear plants?	Beryllium

Which hepatitis B serology markers—HB$_c$Ab IgG, HB$_c$Ab IgM, HB$_e$Ag, HB$_s$Ab IgG, HB$_s$Ag, HBV-DNA— are associated with the following periods?

Window period	HB$_c$Ab IgM
Immunization	HB$_s$Ab IgG
Prior infection	HB$_c$Ab IgG and HB$_s$Ab IgG
Acute infection	HB$_c$Ab IgM, HBV-DNA, HB$_e$Ag, HB$_s$Ag
Chronic infection	HB$_c$Ab IgG, HBV-DNA, HB$_e$Ag, HB$_s$Ag

Name the type of necrosis.

The *most common* form of necrosis; denatured and coagulated proteins in the cytoplasm	Coagulative necrosis
Seen as dead tissue with *coagulative* necrosis	Gangrenous necrosis
Seen as dead tissue with *liquefactive* necrosis?	Liquefaction necrosis
Due to lipase activity and has a *chalky white* appearance	Fat necrosis
Soft, friable, *cottage-cheese* appearing; characteristically seen in *TB*	Caseous necrosis
Histologically resembles *fibrin*	Fibrinoid necrosis

Name two of three enzymes that protect the cell from oxygen-derived free radicals.	Superoxide dismutase, glutathione peroxidase, catalase
What are the rules of 2 for Meckel diverticulum?	2% of population, 2 cm long, 2 feet from ileocecal valve, 2 years old, and 2% of carcinoid tumors
What aneurysm of the circle of Willis is associated with polycystic kidney disease?	Berry aneurysm
A 20-year-old black woman goes to you with nonspecific joint pain, fever, and a malar rash over the bridge of her nose and on her cheeks. This is a classic example of what autoimmune disease? What are three autoantibody tests you could order to make the diagnosis?	SLE; ANA, anti-dsDNA and anti-Sm (anti-Smith)
True or false? Excess lead deposits in the oral cavity.	True. It deposits at the gingivodental line, known as the lead line.
What is the term for increased iron deposition resulting in micronodular cirrhosis, CHF, diabetes, and bronzing of the skin?	Hemochromatosis
What *AR* disorder is due to a deficiency in glycoprotein *IIb-IIIa*, resulting in a defect in *platelet aggregation*?	Glanzmann syndrome
What protein-losing enteropathy has grossly	Ménétrier's disease

enlarged rugal fold in the body and fundus of the stomach in middle-aged males, resulting in decreased acid production and an increased risk of gastric cancer?

What myopathy due to autoantibodies to ACh receptors can present with thymic abnormalities, red cell aplasia, and muscle weakness?

Myasthenia gravis

Which subtype of AML is most commonly associated with Auer rods?

M3 (promyelocytic leukemia)

What condition results from a 46XX karyotype and female internal organs with virilized external genitalia?

Female pseudohermaphrodite

Two weeks after her son has a throat infection, a mother takes the boy to the ER because he has fever, malaise, HTN, dark urine, and periorbital edema. What is your diagnosis?

Poststreptococcal GN

What *X-linked recessive* immune disorder is characterized by *recurrent infections*, severe *thrombocytopenia*, and *eczema*?

Wiskott-Aldrich syndrome

What form of arthritis is associated with calcium pyrophosphate crystals?

Pseudogout

What is the term for excessive production of collagen that flattens out and does not extend beyond the site of the injury?	Hypertrophic scar
What is the term for inflamed, thickened skin on the breast with dimpling associated with cancer?	Peau d'orange
What rare vasculitis has the following characteristics: males aged 40 to 60; affecting *small* arteries and veins; involving *nose*, *sinuses*, *lungs*, and *kidneys*; *C-ANCA* and autoantibodies against *proteinase* 3?	Wegener granulomatosis
What retrovirus is associated with adult T-cell leukemia?	HTLV-1
What disease is seen in children younger than 5 years of age and is characterized by X-linked recessive cardiac myopathies, calf pseudohypertrophy, lordosis, protuberant belly, an increase then a decrease in CPK, and death commonly in the second decade of life?	Duchenne muscular dystrophy
What malignant neoplasm of the bone has a soap bubble appearance on radiograph?	Giant cell bone tumor (osteoclastoma)

What nephritic syndrome has effacement of the epithelial foot processes *without* immune complex deposition?

Minimal change disease

What is the term for tissue-based basophils?

Mast cells

What malignant bone tumor is characterized by Codman triangle (periosteal elevation) on radiograph?

Osteosarcoma

Is splenomegaly *more commonly* associated with intravascular or extravascular hemolysis?

Extravascular hemolysis if it occurs in the spleen; if in the liver, it results in hepatomegaly.

What cancer of the male genitourinary system is associated with osteoblastic bony metastasis?

Prostatic carcinoma

What stromal tumor in males is characterized histologically with crystalloids of Reinke?

Leydig cell tumor

What pulmonary disease, most commonly associated with smoking, results in enlarged, overinflated lungs owing to the destruction of the alveolar walls with diminished elastic recoil?

Emphysema

What factor gets activated in the *intrinsic pathway* of the coagulation cascade? *Extrinsic pathway*?

Factor XII for the **intrinsic**; factor VII for the **extrinsic pathway**

What chronic systemic inflammatory disease commonly seen in women aged 20 to 50 is a progressive, symmetric arthritis affecting the hands, wrists, knees, and ankles that *improves with increased activity*?	Rheumatoid arthritis

Name the following descriptions associated with bacterial endocarditis:

Retinal emboli	Roth spots
***Painful* subcutaneous nodules on fingers and toes**	Osler nodes
***Painless* hyperemic lesions on the palms and soles**	Janeway lesions
What two CD cell surface markers do Reed-Sternberg cells stain positive for?	CD15 and CD30
What two lysosomal storage diseases have *cherry-red spots* on the retina?	Niemann-Pick and Tay-Sachs diseases
True or false? Increased LAP is associated with CML.	False. Increased LAP is seen in stress reactions and helps differentiate benign conditions from CML, which has low LAP levels.
What syndrome has multiple adenomatous colonic polyps and CNS gliomas?	Turcot syndrome

What is the term for a venous embolus in the arterial system?

Paradoxic emboli most commonly enter the arteries through a patent septal defect in the heart.

Are hemorrhagic cerebral infarcts more commonly associated with embolic or thrombotic occlusions?

Embolic

What is the name for the following RBC indices?

> **The coefficient of variation of the RBC volume**

RDW

> **Average mass of the Hgb molecule/RBC**

MCH

> **Average volume of a RBC**

MCV

> **Average Hgb concentration/given volume of packed RBCs**

MCHC

What cardiomyopathy is due to a ventricular outflow obstruction as a result of septal hypertrophy and leads to sudden cardiac death in young athletes?

Hypertrophic cardiomyopathy (hypertrophic subaortic stenosis, or IHSS)

Which HPV serotypes are associated with condyloma acuminatum?

HPV serotypes 6 and 11

Which form of melanoma carries the best prognosis?

Lentigo maligna melanoma

What is the term for an increase in the *number of cells* in a tissue?

Hyperplasia

A 60-year-old man has back pain (compression spinal fracture), hypercalcemia, increased serum protein, Bence-Jones proteinuria, and monoclonal M-spike on serum electrophoresis. What is your diagnosis?	Multiple myeloma
What is the term for pus in the pleural space?	Empyema
What is a flat, circumscribed nonpalpable pigmented change up to 1 cm?	Macule (e.g., a freckle)

Name the macrophage based on its location:

Liver macrophages	Kupffer cells
Bone macrophages	Osteoclasts
Brain macrophages	Microglia
Lung macrophages	Pulmonary alveolar macrophages
Connective tissue macrophages	Histiocytes
Epidermal macrophages	Langerhans cells

What is the term for a large, immature RBC that is spherical, blue, and without a nucleus?	Reticulocyte
What testicular tumor of infancy is characterized by elevated α-fetoprotein levels and Schiller-Duval bodies?	Yolk sac tumor

Starry sky appearance of macrophages is pathognomonic of what lymphoma?

Burkitt lymphoma

In which region of the lung are 75% of the pulmonary infarcts seen?

Lower lobe

For what disease are SS-A(Ro), SS-B(La), and R-ANA diagnostic markers?

Sjögren disease

What HPV serotypes are associated with increased risk of cervical cancer?

HPV serotypes 16, 18, 31, and 33

Do the following structures pick up stain from hematoxylin or eosin?

Nuclei	Hematoxylin
Nucleoli	Hematoxylin
Cytoplasm	Eosin
Collagen	Eosin
RBCs	Eosin
Calcium	Hematoxylin
Bacteria	Hematoxylin
Fibrin	Eosin
Thyroid colloid	Eosin

What commonly encountered overdose produces *headache*, *tinnitus*, respiratory alkalosis, metabolic acidosis, confusion, vomiting, and tachypnea?

ASA (salicylate)

What *AR* syndrome is due to a deficiency of glycoprotein *Ib*, resulting in a defect in *platelet adhesion*?

Bernard-Soulier syndrome

What AD renal disorder is associated with mutations of the PKD 1 gene on chromosome 16 and berry aneurysms in the circle of Willis and presents in the fifth decade with abdominal masses, flank pain, hematuria, HTN, and renal insufficiency?

Adult polycystic kidney disease

Based on the following information, is the renal transplantation rejection acute, chronic, or hyperacute?

Months to years after transplantation; gradual onset of HTN, oliguria, and azotemia; seen as intimal fibrosis of the blood vessels and interstitial lymphocytes

Chronic rejection

Immediately after transplantation; seen as a neutrophilic vasculitis with thrombosis

Hyperacute rejection

Weeks to months after transplantation; abrupt onset of oliguria and azotemia; seen as neutrophilic vasculitis and interstitial lymphocytes

Acute rejection

What type of collagen is abnormal in patients with osteogenesis imperfecta?

Type I (makes sense, since they have a predisposition for fractures and type I collagen is associated with bones and tendons)

What *coronary artery* vasculitis is seen in *Japanese* infants and children less than *4 years old* with acute febrile illness, conjunctivitis, maculopapular rash, and lymphadenopathy?

Kawasaki disease

What disease has autoantibodies to IgG, occurs in women more than men, and includes exophthalmos, pretibial myxedema, nervousness, heart palpitations, and fatigue?

Graves disease

What condition is defined by both testicular and ovarian tissues in one individual?

True hermaphrodism

A mother takes her 2-week-old infant to the ER because the baby regurgitates and vomits after eating and has peristaltic waves visible on the abdomen and a palpable mass in the right upper quadrant. What is your diagnosis?

Pyloric stenosis

What variant of polyarteritis nodosa is associated with bronchial asthma, granulomas, and eosinophilia?

Churg-Strauss syndrome

What component of the basement membrane binds to collagen type IV and heparin sulfate and is a cell surface receptor?	Laminin
What B-cell neoplasm is seen in males with massive splenomegaly, produces dry tap on bone marrow aspirations, and stains positive for tartrate-resistant acid phosphatase (TRAP)?	Hairy cell leukemia
What form of nephritic syndrome is associated with celiac sprue and Henoch-Schönlein purpura?	IgA nephropathy
What syndrome is characterized by embryologic failure of the third and fourth *pharyngeal pouches* resulting in *hypocalcemia, tetany,* and T-cell deficiency?	DiGeorge syndrome
What is the treatment for physiologic jaundice of newborns?	Phototherapy
How many months in how many years must a person cough with copious sputum production for the diagnosis of chronic bronchitis to be made?	**3 months** of symptoms in **2 consecutive years**
What chronic inflammatory WBC is associated with IgE-mediated allergic reactions and parasitic infections?	Eosinophils

What *AD* syndrome produces hamartomatous polyps in the small intestine and pigmentation of the lips and oral mucosa?

Peutz-Jeghers syndrome

What is the term for formation of a stable fibrin–platelet plug to stop bleeding?

Hemostasis

True or false? All of the following are risk factors for breast cancer: early menses, late menopause, history of breast cancer, obesity, and multiparity.

False. All **except multiparity** are risk factors for breast cancer. **Nulli**parity, increasing age, and family history in first-degree relative are also risk factors. Memorize this list!

Is jugular venous distention a presentation of isolated left or right heart failure?

Right-sided

Name the hepatitis virus based on the following information.

Small circular RNA virus with defective envelope

Hepatitis D

Enveloped RNA flavivirus

Hepatitis C

Naked capsid RNA calicivirus

Hepatitis E

Enveloped DNA hepadnavirus

Hepatitis B

Naked capsid RNA picornavirus

Hepatitis A

What AR disease involves a decreased amount of sphingomyelinase, massive organomegaly, zebra bodies, and foamy histiocytes and is associated with chromosome 11p?	Niemann-Pick disease
What is the term for hypoperfusion of an area involving only the inner layers?	Mural infarct
What are the three causes of normochromic normocytic anemia with a normal MCV and a low reticulocyte count?	Marrow failure, cancer, and leukemia
Notching of the ribs, seen on chest radiograph in patients with postductal coarctation of the aorta, is due to collateralization of what arteries?	Dilation of the **internal mammary arteries** results in erosions on the inner surface of the ribs and is seen as notching.
What is the physiologic storage form of iron?	Ferritin
What is the term for occlusion of a blood vessel due to an intravascular mass that has been carried downstream?	Embolism
What *AR* disorder of *copper metabolism* can be characterized by Kayser-Fleischer rings, decreased ceruloplasmin levels, and increased urinary copper excretion and tissue copper levels?	Wilson disease. (Remember, patients commonly present with psychiatric manifestations and movement disorders but may be asymptomatic.)

Name the cancer associated with the following oncogenes. (Some may have more than one answer)

c-myc	Burkitt lymphoma
L-myc	Small cell cancer of the lung
hst-1 and int-2	Melanoma, cancer of the stomach and bladder
ret	MEN II and III syndromes
Ki-ras	Pancreas and colon
cyclin D	Mantle cell lymphoma
N-myc	Neuroblastoma
CDK4	Melanoma
abl	CML and ALL
hst-1, int-2, erb-2, and erb-3	Breast cancer
sis	Astrocytoma
Ki-ras and erb-2	Lung cancer
erb-1	Squamous cell carcinoma of the lung
What *AD* GI neoplasia produces multiple adenomatous polyps, osteomas, fibromas, and epidural inclusion cysts?	Gardner syndrome
What disease involves microcephaly, mental retardation, cleft lip or palate, and dextrocardia?	Patau syndrome (trisomy 13)

What type of GN occurs most commonly in children after a pharyngeal or skin infection; is immune complex–mediated; and is seen as lumpy-bumpy subepithelial deposits?

Postinfectious GN

What are the three most common sites for left-sided heart embolisms to metastasize?

Brain, spleen, and kidney

With what two pathologies is a honeycomb lung associated?

Asbestosis and silicosis

What AD disorder due to a mutation in fibroblast growth factor receptor 3 results in normal-size vertebral column and skull and short, thick extremities?

Achondroplasia

8 ___ Power Review

BUZZWORDS

Calf pseudohypertrophy	Duchenne muscular dystrophy
Kayser-Fleischer rings	Wilson disease
Aschoff bodies	Rheumatic fever
Curschmann spirals	Bronchial asthma (whorled mucous plugs)
Charcot-Leyden crystals	Bronchial asthma (eosinophil membranes)
Keratin pearls	Squamous cell carcinoma
Bence-Jones proteinuria	Multiple myeloma
Russell bodies	Multiple myeloma
WBCs in the urine	Acute cystitis
RBCs in the urine	Bladder carcinoma
RBC casts in the urine	Acute glomerulonephritis
WBC casts in the urine	Acute pyelonephritis
Renal epithelial casts in the urine	Acute toxic or viral nephrosis
Waxy casts	Chronic end-stage renal disease
Signet ring cells	Gastric carcinoma

Heinz bodies	G-6-PD deficiency
Mallory bodies	Chronic alcoholic
Auer rods	AML-M3
Starry sky pattern	Burkitt lymphoma
Birbeck granules	Histiocytosis X
Reed-Sternberg cells	Hodgkin lymphoma
Call-Exner bodies	Granulosa/thecal cell tumor of the ovary
Cowdry type A bodies	Herpesvirus
Orphan Annie cells	Papillary carcinoma of the ovary
Streaky ovaries	Turner syndrome
Blue-domed cysts	Fibrocystic change of the breast
Reinke crystals	Leydig cell tumor
Schiller-Duval bodies	Yolk sac tumor
Codman triangle on radiograph	Osteosarcoma
Councilman bodies	Toxic or viral hepatitis
Blue sclera	Osteogenesis imperfecta
Soap bubble appearance on radiograph	Giant cell tumor of the bone
Pseudorosettes	Ewing sarcoma
Neurofibrillary tangles	Alzheimer disease
Homer-Wright rosettes	Neuroblastoma
Lewy bodies	Parkinson disease

Lucid interval	Epidural hematoma
Bloody tap on lumbar puncture	Subarachnoid hemorrhage
Pseudopalisades	Glioblastoma multiforme
Senile plaques	Alzheimer disease
Café-au-lait spot on the skin	Neurofibromatosis

MOST COMMON

Name the most common cause.

Blindness worldwide	*Chlamydia trachomatis*
Blindness in the United States	Diabetes mellitus
Dementia in persons aged 60 to 90 years	Alzheimer disease

Name the most common type.

Learning disability	Dyslexia
Mental retardation	Fetal alcohol syndrome
Phobia	Stage fright (discrete performance anxiety)
Psychiatric disorder in women of all ages	Anxiety disorders; for men it is substance abuse.
***Specific* phobia**	Public speaking (Remember: stage fright)

Name the most common cause.

Chronic pancreatitis	Alcohol abuse

Infectious pancreatitis	Mumps
Insomnia	Depression
Hospitalization in children younger than 1 year of age	RSV
Croup	Parainfluenza virus
A cold in the winter and summer	Coronavirus
A cold in the spring and fall	Rhinovirus
Which virus is the MCC of a cold in the summer and fall? Winter and spring?	Rhinoviruses for summer and fall; coronaviruses for winter and spring

Name the most common type or cause.

Restrictive cardiomyopathy	Amyloidosis
Death in the United States	Ischemic heart disease (MIs)
Sudden cardiac death	Ventricular fibrillation (V fib)
Right heart failure	Left heart failure
Childhood heart disease in the United States	Congenital heart disease
Cyanotic heart disease	Tetralogy of Fallot
Subacute bacterial endocarditis	*Streptococcus viridans*
Acute bacterial endocarditis	*Staphylococcus aureus*

Viral pneumonia leading to death	RSV
Infection in a patient on a ventilator	*Pseudomonas aeruginosa*
Bronchiolitis in children	RSV
Pulmonary HTN in children	VSD
Reversible HTN in the United States	Alcohol abuse
Spontaneous pneumothorax	Emphysematous bleb
Nonorganic pneumoconiosis	Asbestosis
Cellular injury	Hypoxia
Hypoxia	Ischemia
Lobar pneumonia	*Streptococcus pneumoniae*
Lung abscess	Aspiration
Cirrhosis in the United States	Alcohol consumption
Nephrotic syndrome	Membranoproliferative glomerulonephritis (MGN)
Nephrotic syndrome in children	Lipoid nephrosis
Liver transplantation in adults	Alcoholic cirrhosis
UTIs	Escherichia coli
Urinary tract obstruction	BPH

Painless hematuria	Renal cell carcinoma
Hematuria	Infection
GN in the world	IgA nephropathy
Nephritic syndrome in children	Minimal change disease
Nephritic syndrome in adults	MGN
Acute renal failure in the United States	Acute tubular necrosis
Acute tubular necrosis	Ischemic
Diarrhea in children	Rotavirus
Intestinal obstructions in adults	Adhesions and hernias
Neonatal bowel obstruction	Hirschsprung disease
Rectal bleeding	Diverticulosis
Mallory-Weiss syndrome	Alcoholism
Anovulation	Polycystic ovaries
Breast lump in females	Fibrocystic change of the breast
Hematologic cause of papillary necrosis	Sickle cell disease
Panhypopituitarism	Sheehan syndrome
Cushing syndrome	Pituitary adenoma
Noniatrogenic hypothyroidism in the United States	Hashimoto thyroiditis

Hypothyroidism in the United States	Iatrogenesis
Pyogenic osteomyelitis	*Staphylococcus aureus*
Neonatal septicemia and meningitis	*Streptococcus agalactiae* (Group B *Streptococcus*, or GBS)
Sinusitis and otitis media in children	*Pneumococcus*
Meningitis in adults	*Pneumococcus*
Meningitis in renal transplantation patients	*Listeria monocytogenes*
Infantile bacterial diarrhea	Enteropathogenic *Escherichia coli* (Rotavirus is the MCC overall.)
Infantile diarrhea	Rotavirus
Chancre	*Haemophilus ducreyi*
Urethritis in a young, newly sexually active individual	*Staphylococcus saprophyticus*
Cystitis	*Escherichia coli*
Erysipelas	*Streptococcus pyogenes*
Chronic metal poisoning	Lead
***Acute* metal poisoning in the United States**	Arsenic

Name the MCC of death.

In neonates	Neonatal respiratory distress syndrome (NRDS)
In SLE	Renal failure

In diabetic individuals	MI
In patients with cystic fibrosis	Pulmonary infections
What is the MCC of death in the United States?	Heart disease
What is the second leading cause of death in the United States?	Cancer
What is the MCC of death in children aged 1 to 14 in the United States?	Accidents
What is the second leading cause of death in children aged 1 to 14 in the United States?	Cancer
What is the MCC of cancer *mortality* in males and females?	Lung cancer
What is the *second* leading cause of cancer *deaths* in males? In females?	For males it's prostate cancer, and for females it's breast cancer.
What is the MCC of death in black males aged 15 to 24?	Homicide. It is also the leading cause of death in black females aged 15 to 24.
What are the two MCC of acute epididymitis in males?	
Less than 35 years old	*Neisseria gonorrhoeae* and *Chlamydia trachomatis*
More than 35 years old	*Escherichia coli* and *Pseudomonas* sp.
What is the most common causative organism of *acne vulgaris*?	*Propionibacterium acnes*

What is the MCC of viral conjunctivitis?	Adenovirus

What is the MCC of the following endocarditis scenarios?

Post dental work	*Streptococcus viridans*
Following biliary infections	*Enterococcus faecalis*
Non–IV drug user	*Staphylococcus aureus*

Name the MCC.

Epiglottitis in an unvaccinated child	*Haemophilus influenzae* type B
Pneumonia in adults	*Streptococcus pneumoniae*
Pneumonia in a neutropenic burn patient	*Pseudomonas* sp.
Pneumonia in a patient with atypical bird exposure and hepatitis	*Chlamydia psittaci*
Walking pneumonia, seen in teens and military recruits	*Mycoplasma pneumoniae*
Aspiration pneumonia in an alcoholic	*Klebsiella pneumoniae*
Pneumonia in an HIV-positive patient with CD4 less than 200	*Pneumocystis carinii*

What is the MCC of the following meningitides?

In patients who have AIDS or are immunocompromised	*Cryptococcus*

In military recruits	*Neisseria meningitides*
In those 12 months to 6 years of age	*Haemophilus influenzae* type B
In neonates to 3 months of age	*Streptococcus agalactiae* and *Escherichia coli*
In adults	*Streptococcus pneumoniae*
In renal transplant patients	*Listeria monocytogenes*

What is the most common one?

Helminthic parasite worldwide	*Ascaris lumbricoides*
Helminth parasitic infection in the United States	*Enterobius vermicularis*
Form of necrosis	Coagulative
Organism that causes pyelonephritis	*Escherichia coli*
Congenital cardiac anomaly	VSD
Cardiac anomaly in children	PDA
Complication of PDA	Subacute bacterial endocarditis
Congenital heart defect in adults	ASD
Type of ASD	Ostium secundum defects
Vasculitis	Temporal arteritis
Form of vasculitis	Temporal arteritis

Cardiac tumor	Left atrial myxoma
Cardiac tumor of infancy	Rhabdomyoma
Cardiac pathology in patients with SLE	Libman-Sacks endocarditis
Cardiac anomaly in Turner syndrome	Coarctation of the aorta
Valve abnormality associated with rheumatic fever	Mitral valve stenosis
Viral cause of myocarditis	Coxsackie B
Primary lung cancer	Adenocarcinoma
Primary malignant tumor of the lungs	Adenocarcinoma (30% to 35%)
Neoplastic tumor in the lungs	Metastatic carcinomas
Bladder tumor	Transitional cell carcinoma
Renal calculus type	Calcium oxylate
Kidney stone type	Calcium oxalate
Solid tumor in children	Neuroblastoma
Renal pathology in patients with SLE	Diffuse proliferative GN
Cancer of the esophagus in the world	Squamous cell carcinoma
Esophageal cancer in the United States	Adenocarcinoma (because of Barrett esophagus)
Malignant tumor of the esophagus	Squamous cell carcinoma

Benign GI tumor	Leiomyoma
Site of ischemia in the GI tract	Splenic flexure
Type of PUD	Duodenal ulcers (4 times as common as gastric)
Location of a duodenal ulcer	Anterior wall of the first part of the duodenum
Location of a gastric ulcer	Lesser curvature of the antrum of the stomach
Site for carcinoid tumors	Appendix (second is terminal ileum)
Site for colonic diverticula	Sigmoid colon
Site of Crohn disease	Terminal ileum
Site of ulcerative colitis	Rectum
Site of pancreatic cancer	Head of the pancreas
Pancreatic islet cell tumor	Insulinoma
Stone type associated with cholecystitis	Mixed (both cholesterol and calcium)
Liver tumor	Metastatic carcinoma
Primary malignant tumor in the liver	Hepatocellular carcinoma
Primary tumor of the liver	Hemangioma (benign)
Organism associated with liver abscesses	*Entamoeba histolytica*
Renal cell cancer type	Clear cell

Esophageal carcinoma	Squamous cell carcinoma
Solid tumor in the body	Nephroblastoma
Malignancy in children	ALL
Lymph node affected in non-Hodgkin lymphoma	Periaortic lymph nodes
Subtype of Hodgkin lymphoma	Nodular sclerosis
Thyroid cancer	Papillary carcinoma
Thyroid adenoma	Follicular adenoma
Malignant thyroid tumor	Papillary carcinoma of the thyroid
Pituitary tumor	Chromophobe adenoma
Pituitary adenoma	Prolactinoma
Tumor arising within the bone	Multiple myeloma
Tumor on sun-exposed sites	Basal cell carcinoma
Malignant germ cell tumor in women	Choriocarcinoma
Primary malignant tumor of the ovary	Serocystadenocarcinoma
Malignant tumor in women	Breast
Cancer of the vulva	Squamous cell carcinoma
Primary malignant tumor of the female genital tract in the world	Cervical neoplasia

Primary malignant tumor of the female genital tract in the United States	Adenocarcinoma of the cervix
Tumor of the female genitourinary tract	Leiomyoma
Benign tumor of the ovary	Serocystadenoma
Benign tumor of the breast	Fibroadenoma
Benign breast tumor in females less than 35 years old	Fibroadenoma
Histologic variant of breast cancer	Infiltrating ductal carcinoma
Benign lesion that affects the breast	Fibrocystic change of the breast
Malignant tumor of the breast	Invasive ductal carcinoma
Female genital tract malignancy resulting in death	Ovarian cancer
Malignancy of the female genital tract	Endometrial cancer
Tumor of the female genital tract	Leiomyoma (fibroids)
Benign ovarian tumor	Cystadenoma
Malignant carcinoma of the ovaries	Cystadenocarcinoma
Stromal tumor of the ovary	Ovarian fibroma

Germ cell tumor of the ovary	Dysgerminoma
Tumor in men aged 15 to 35	Testicular tumors
Testicular tumor in men over 50 years old	Testicular lymphoma
Germ cell tumor in men	Seminoma
Testicular tumor in infants and children	Yolk sac tumor
Germ cell tumor in boys	Yolk sac tumor
Malignant tumor in the bone of teenagers	Osteosarcoma
Intraspinal tumor	Ependymoma
Eye tumor in children	Retinoblastoma
Organ involved in amyloidosis	Kidney
Complication of nasogastric tube feeding	Aspiration pneumonia
Acquired GI emergency of infancy	Necrotizing enterocolitis
Organism associated with mastitis	*Staphylococcus aureus*
Tumor in individuals exposed to asbestos	Bronchogenic carcinoma
Proliferative abnormality of an internal organ	BPH
Inflammatory arthritis	Rheumatoid arthritis

Form of muscular dystrophy	Duchenne muscular dystrophy
Joint affected in pseudogout	Knee
Route for infectious arthritis	Hematogenous
Form of arthritis	Osteoarthritis
Route of spread in pyogenic osteomyelitis	Hematogenous
Bone disorder in the United States	Osteoporosis
Primary tumor metastasis to the bone	Breast
Bone tumor	Metastatic
Neurotransmitter in the brain	GABA, quantitatively
Site of a cerebral infarct	Middle cerebral artery
Primary CNS tumor in adults	Glioblastoma multiforme
Primary CNS tumor in children	Medulla blastoma
Brain tumor	Metastatic
Primary CNS tumor	Glioblastoma multiforme
Intramedullary spinal cord tumor in adults	Ependymoma
Location of ependymomas in children	In children, the fourth ventricle; in adults, the lateral ventricle or spinal cord

Melanoma in dark-skinned persons	Acral-lentiginous melanoma
Type of melanoma	Superficial spreading melanoma
Skin tumor in the United States	Basal cell carcinoma
Site of congenital diaphragmatic hernias	Left posterolateral side of the diaphragm, usually resulting in pulmonary hypoplasia.
Type of hernia seen in males more than 50 years old	Direct; in males less than 50 years old indirect hernias are the most common type.
Sites for abdominal aorta aneurysm	Between the renal arteries and at the bifurcation of the abdominal aorta
Site for atherosclerotic plaques in the abdominal aorta	The bifurcation of the abdominal aorta
Site for an ectopic abdominal pregnancy	The rectouterine pouch (of Douglas)
What is the most common site for implantation of the blastocyst?	On the superior body of the posterior wall of the uterus
Where is the most frequent site of ectopic pregnancy?	Ampulla of the fallopian tube
What is the most common diagnosis made (or missed!) resulting in a malpractice suit?	Breast cancer
What is the most common serotype of enterohemorrhagic *Escherichia coli*?	0157:H7
What is the most common circulation Ig in the plasma?	IgG

What is the most common cancer diagnosed in men? In women?	In men it is prostate cancer, and in women it is breast cancer.
What is the second most common cancer diagnosed in both males and females?	Lung and bronchus cancer
What are the two leading causes of cancer-related death in men?	Prostate and lung cancer, respectively
What are the two leading causes of cancer-related death in women?	Breast and lung cancer, respectively.
What is the most common primary diagnosis resulting in an office visit for males? For females?	For males, HTN; for females, pregnancy.
What is the most common disease or infection reported to the CDC?	Chlamydia; gonorrhea is second (Remember, it is mandatory to report STDs to the CDC.)
What is the most common STD?	HPV
Name the most common reported STD.	
In females	Chlamydia
In males	Gonorrhea
What is the most common sexual assault?	Pedophilia
What is the most common form of elderly abuse?	Nearly 50% of all reported cases of elderly abuse are due to neglect. Physical, psychological, and financial are other forms of elderly abuse with an overall prevalence rate of 5% to 10%.

What is the most common complement deficiency?

C_2 deficiency

What is the most common organ involved in amyloidosis?

Kidney

What is the most common form of non-Hodgkin lymphoma in the United States?

Follicular lymphoma

In which quadrant is breast cancer most commonly found?

Upper outer quadrant (left more than right)

What is the most common cardiac tumor? In what chamber does it most commonly arise?

90% of benign myxomas arise within the left atrium near the fossa ovalis.

What cerebral lobes are most commonly affected in herpes encephalitis?

Temporal lobes

What is the most common condition leading to an intracerebral bleed?

HTN

What carpal bone is most commonly fractured? Dislocated?

The scaphoid is the most commonly fractured and the lunate is the most commonly dislocated.

What is the costliest health care problem in the United States?

Alcohol and its related problems cost the country approximately $100 billion a year.

What is the most abused drug across all age groups?

Alcohol. Nearly 10% of adults have a problem with alcohol.

What are the two most common chains of the TCR?

α-and β-chains are on most T cells.

What is the most common form of inherited dwarfism?	Achondroplasia
What is the most common lethal AR disorder affecting white Americans?	Cystic fibrosis
What is the most common genetic cause of mental retardation?	Down syndrome (it is slightly more common than fragile X syndrome.)
What is the most common chromosomal abnormality associated with CLL?	Trisomy 12 (nearly 50% of patients with CLL have abnormal karyotypes.)

Name the most common one.

Chromosomal disorder	Down syndrome (trisomy 21)
Heart defect in Down syndrome	Endocardial cushion defect
Chromosomal disorder involving sex chromosomes	Klinefelter syndrome

CHROMOSOMES

Name the associated chromosomal translocation.

CML	Chromosome 9,22 (Philadelphia chromosome)
Ewing sarcoma	Chromosome 11,22
Adult familial polyposis	Chromosome 5,21
Burkitt lymphoma	Chromosome 8,14
Acute promyelocytic leukemia (M3)	Chromosome 15,17

M3 AML	Chromosome 15,17
Follicular lymphoma	Chromosome 14,18

Name the associated chromosome.

Cri-du-chat	Chromosome 5p
Patau syndrome	Chromosome 13
Huntington disease	Chromosome 4p
Familial hypercholesterolemia	Chromosome 19
Gaucher disease	Chromosome 1
Niemann-Pick disease	Chromosome 11p
Tay-Sachs disease	Chromosome 15q
Cystic fibrosis	Chromosome 7
Albinism	Chromosome 11p
Chronic lymphocytic leukemia (CLL)	Chromosome 12
Marfan disease	Chromosome 15
Neurofibromatosis type 1	Chromosome 17
Neurofibromatosis type 2	Chromosome 22q
Down syndrome	Chromosome 21
Edward syndrome	Chromosome 18
von Hippel-Lindau disease	Chromosome 3p

What is the most common chromosomal disorder?	Down syndrome

What is the MCC of *inherited* mental retardation?	Down syndrome
What is the most common lysosomal storage disorder?	Gaucher disease
What chromosome is mutant in patients with cystic fibrosis?	Patients with cystic fibrosis have a mutation in the chloride channel protein in the CFTR gene on chromosome 7.
Familial hypercholesteremia is due to a mutation in the LDL receptor gene. What chromosome carries it?	Chromosome 19
What chromosome is associated with the *AR* form of SCID?	Chromosome 20q (deficiency in adenosine deaminase)
On what chromosome is the adenomatous polyposis coli gene?	Chromosome 5q21

VITAMINS AND MINERALS

What mineral is associated with impaired glucose tolerance?	Chromium (Cr)
What mineral is associated with hypothyroidism?	Iodine (I)
What mineral is an important component of the enzyme xanthine oxidase?	Molybdenum (Mb)
What vitamin deficiency produces angular stomatitis, glossitis, and cheilosis?	Riboflavin (B_2) deficiency

What vitamin is a component of the coenzyme thiamine pyrophosphate (TPP) ?

Thymine (B_1)

Avidin decreases the absorption of what vitamin?

Biotin. Avidin is found in raw egg whites.

What are the four Ds of niacin deficiency?

1. Diarrhea
2. Dermatitis
3. Dementia
4. Death

What mineral is an important component of glutathione peroxidase?

Selenium (Se)

What mineral deficiency in children is associated with poor growth and impaired sexual development?

Zinc (Zn) deficiency

What mineral, via excessive depositions in the liver, causes hemochromatosis?

Iron (Fe)

What vitamin is needed for the production of heme?

Pyridoxine (B_6)

What vitamin is a component of the enzymes fatty acid synthase and acyl CoA?

Pantothenic acid

What vitamin deficiency produces homocystinuria and methylmalonic aciduria?

Cyanocobalamin (B_{12}) deficiency (Folic acid deficiency has only homocystinuria as a sign.)

What vitamin deficiency is evidenced by poor wound healing, loose teeth, bleeding gums, petechiae, and ecchymosis?

Ascorbic acid (vitamin C) deficiency (These are the signs of scurvy.)

What vitamin is given as prophylactic treatment for patients with alcoholism?	Thiamine (B_1), to prevent Wernicke encephalopathy and Korsakoff encephalopathy
What are the three carboxylase enzymes that require biotin?	Pyruvate, acetyl CoA, and propionyl CoA carboxylase
What vitamin requires IF for absorption?	Cyanocobalamin (B_{12})
What mineral is a component of cytochrome a/a_3?	Copper
Leukopenia, neutropenia, and mental deterioration are signs of what mineral deficiency?	Copper
What vitamin deficiency causes a glove-and-stocking neuropathy seen in alcoholics?	Pyridoxine (B_6) deficiency
What mineral deficiency involves blood vessel fragility?	Copper deficiency
Megaloblastic anemia and thrombocytopenia are signs of what vitamin deficiency?	Folic acid deficiency
What vitamin deficiency can result in high-output cardiac failure?	Thiamine

ANTIDOTES

Name the antidote.

Carbon monoxide (CO)	Oxygen

Mercury	Dimercaprol, penicillamine
Isoniazid	Pyridoxine
Atropine	Physostigmine
Arsenic	Dimercaprol, D-penicillamine
Digoxin	Antidigoxin Fab fragments
Gold	Dimercaprol
Ethylene glycol	Ethyl alcohol
Opioids	Naloxone, naltrexone
Organophosphates	Atropine, 2-PAM (pralidoxime)
Warfarin	Vitamin K
Copper	D-Penicillamine
Heparin	Protamine sulfate
Iron	Deferoxamine, penicillamine
Cyanide	Amyl nitrate, sodium nitrate, or sodium thiosulfate
Methyl alcohol	Ethyl alcohol
Acetaminophen	N-Acetylcysteine
Nitrates	Methylene blue
Lead	Penicillamine, EDTA (calcium disodium edetate), or dimercaprol
Benzodiazepines	Flumazenil
AChE inhibitors	Atropine with pralidoxime
Anticholinergics	Physostigmine

A known IV drug abuser goes to the ER with respiratory depression and pinpoint pupils and in a semicomatose state. What overdose do you suspect, and what agent will you give to reverse its effects?

The triad of respiratory depression, pinpoint pupils, and coma in an IV drug abuser suggests opioid overdose (e.g., heroin), and you should give naloxone.

Cherry red intoxication is associated with what form of poisoning?

CO

What toxicities are caused by the following agents?

Occupational nitrous oxide exposure

Anemia

Methoxyflurane

Nephrotoxicity

Halothane

Hepatitis, with or without necrosis

What are the first signs of overdose from phenobarbitals?

Nystagmus and ataxia

What are the three signs of morphine overdose?

Pinpoint pupils, decreased respiratory rate, and coma

What is the major pulmonary side effect of μ-activators?

Respiratory depression

What are the two side effects of opioids to which the user will not develop tolerance?

Constipation and miosis

Appendix: Formulas and Equations

CHAPTER 3, BIOCHEMISTRY

PROTEINS AND ENZYMES

Rate of Reaction Rules

If conc. of S $>>$ K_m, then $V_o = V_{max}$
If conc. of S $=$ K_m, then $V_o = V_{max}/2$
If conc. of S $<<$ K_m, then $V_o = (V_{max} \times S)/Km$

ENERGY METABOLISM

Metabolism Rules and Facts

Well-fed (absorptive) state = storage
Postabsorptive state = fasting
Insulin = storage
Glucagon and epinephrine = fasting and markedly increased in starvation
Prolonged fast = starvation

TCA CYCLE: OXIDATIVE PHOSPHORYLATION

TCA Rules and Hints

(aerobic) ATPs/glucose in
Glycolysis = 8 ATPs
Pyruvate dehydrogenase = 6 ATPs
TCA cycle = 24 ATPs
Total/glucose = 38 ATPs

CHAPTER 5, PHYSIOLOGY

GENERAL TOPICS

Body compartment rules

1. Ingest/infuse = increased volume
2a. Hypotonic = low sodium

2b. Hypertonic = high sodium
2c. Isotonic = no change in sodium
 3. Hydration is related to ECF volume status; ICF changes are *compensations* to ECF.
 4. Fluid shifts are *compensations* to changes in solute concentrations in the ECF.

ADH, Aldosterone, Osmolarity, Tonicity

Aldosterone regulates volume = osmolarity
ADH regulates sodium concentrations = tonicity

Driving Force Rules

Equation: DF = Em − Ex
 1. If DF is positive, force is *from* **inside** *to* **outside** the cell.
 2. If DF is negative, force is *from* **outside** into the cell.
 3. If DF is zero, force is at **equilibrium.**

Na$^+$/K$^+$ effects on cell membranes

Na$^+$ = **action potential**
K$^+$ = **resting membrane potential**

CARDIOLOGY AND CIRCULATION

Cardiology Equations and Formulas

$$V = 1/A$$

where V = velocity and A = area.

$$Q = P1 − P2/R$$

where Q = flow, P1 = pressure upstream, P2 = pressure downstream, and R = resistance of the vessel.

$$C = (V1 − V2)/(P1 − P2)$$

where C = compliance.

MAP   = **2/3 diastolic pressure + 1/3 systolic pressure**
          = **(Pulse Pressure/3) + diastolic pressure**
          = **cardiac output × TPR**

$$EF = SV/EDV$$

where EF = ejection fraction, SV = stroke volume, and EDV = end diastolic volume.

$$SV = EDV - ESV$$

where ESV = end systolic volume

PULMONARY

Pulmonary Equations and Concepts

$$Ve = V_T \times f$$

where Ve = total ventilation, V_T = tidal volume, and f = respiratory rate.

$$C = (V1 - V2)/(P1 - P2)$$

where C = compliance
Change in volume
Change in pressure

Ventilation–Perfusion Relationships (V/Q)

Apex: Least ventilated and **least** perfused
: Ventilation exceeds blood flow, resulting in **overinflation**.
: V/Q ratio > 0.8
Base: Most ventilated and **most** perfused
: Blood flow exceeds O_2 delivery, resulting in **underinflation**.
: V/Q ratio < 0.8

Normal intra-alveolar total pressure = 140 mm Hg

$$PAO_2 = 100 \text{ mm Hg}$$

$$PaCO_2 = 40 \text{ mm Hg}$$

Normal beginning pulmonary capillary contents

$$PaO_2 = 40 \text{ mm Hg}$$

$$PaCO_2 = 47 \text{ mm Hg}$$

PO_2 (A − a) difference = 100 − 40 = 60 mm Hg gradient
(large gradient, low solubility)

PCO_2 (A − a) difference = 47 − 40 = 7 mm Hg gradient
(low gradient, high solubility)

ADH, OSMOLARITY, ACID-BASE, AND THE KIDNEY

Renal Equations and Concepts

$$\text{Filtration fraction: FF} = GFR/RPF$$
$$= Cin/Cpah \ (C = \text{clearance})$$

$$\text{Resistance in a series: } Rt = R1 + R2 + R3 + \ldots$$

$$\text{Resistance in parallel: } Rt = 1/R1 + 1/R2 + 1/R3 + \ldots$$

$$\text{Filtered load} = GFR \times (Px)$$

where Px = concentration of a substance in plasma

$$\text{Tubular secreted} = \text{excreted} - \text{filtered}$$

$$\text{Tubular excreted} = \text{secretion} + \text{filtered}$$

$$\text{Reabsorption} = \text{filtration} - \text{excretion}$$

$$\text{Clearance} = ([Ux] \times V)/(Px)$$

where Ux = urine concentration and V = urine flow rate.

Renal blood flow = ERPF/1-Hct

Acid-Base Rules

Follow these rules when evaluating A-B disturbances:
1. Check the pH; is it acidotic or alkalotic?
2. Check CO_2. If increased, acidotic; if decreased, alkalotic.
3. Check HCO_3^-. If decreased, acidotic; if increased, alkalotic.

When evaluating acidosis:
1. pH low = acidosis.
2. CO_2 increased = respiratory component.
3. No change in CO_2 = metabolic component.
4. CO_2 increased and HCO_3^- depressed = mixed picture.

When evaluating alkalosis:
1. pH high = alkalosis.
2. CO_2 decreased = respiratory component.
3. No change in CO_2 = metabolic component.
4. CO_2 decreased and HCO_3^- increased = mixed picture.

Renal compensation for acidosis:
For every HCO_3^- produced by the kidney, one H^+ will be excreted in the urine.

Renal compensation for alkalosis:

For every H^+ produced by the kidney, one HCO_3^- will be excreted in the urine.

CHAPTER 6, PHARMACOLOGY

KINETICS AND DYNAMICS

Pharmacology Equations

$$LD = Vd \times Css$$

where LD = loading dose, Vd = volume of distribution, and Css = plasma at steady state.

$$\mathbf{CL = k \times Vd}$$

where CL = clearance and k = elimination rate constant.

$$\mathbf{k0 = CL \times Css}$$

where k0 = infusion rate.

$$\mathbf{Vd = dose/C0}$$

where C0 = plasma concentration at zero time.

$$\mathbf{t_{1/2} = (0.7 \times Vd)/CL = 0.7/k}$$

where $t_{1/2}$ = elimination half-life.

Bibliography

Barr ML, Kiernan JA: *The Human Nervous System: An Anatomical Viewpoint.* Philadelphia, JB Lippincott, 1993.

Bates B: *A Guide to Physical Examination and History Taking,* 6th ed. Philadelphia, JB Lippincott, 1991.

Benjamini E, Leskowitz S: *Immunology: A Short Course,* 2nd ed. New York, Willey-Liss, 1991.

Berkow R, Fletcher AJ (eds): *Merck Manual of Diagnosis and Therapy,* 16th ed. Rahway, NJ, Merck, 1992.

Champe PC, Harvey RA: *Biochemistry,* 2nd ed. Philadelphia, JB Lippincott, 1994.

Christensen JB: Study Outline for Gross Anatomy, 3rd ed. St. George's University School of Medicine, 1990.

Christensen JB, Telford IR: *Synopsis of Gross Anatomy,* 5th ed. Philadelphia, JB Lippincott, 1988.

Edwards CRW, Boucher IAD (eds): *Davison's Principles and Practices of Medicine,* 16th ed. New York, Churchill Livingstone, 1994.

Fadem B: *Behavioral Science.* Baltimore, Williams & Wilkins, 1991.

Felten DL, Felten SY: *A Regional Overview of Functional Neuroanatomy.* Study outline. Rochester, NY, University of Rochester School of Medicine.

Ganong WF: *A Review of Medical Physiology.* East Norwalk, CT, Appleton & Lange, 1993.

Gartner LP, Hyatt JL: *Color Atlas of Histology.* Baltimore, Williams & Wilkins, 1990.

Guyton AC: *Textbook of Medical Physiology,* 8th ed. Philadelphia, WB Saunders, 1991.

Haines DE: *Neuroanatomy: An Atlas of Structures, Sections and Systems.* Baltimore, Williams & Wilkins, 1990.

Kandel ER, Schwartz JH, Jessel TM: *Principles of Neuroscience,* 3rd ed. East Norwalk, CT, Appleton & Lange, 1991.

Kaplan Medical: *USMLE Step 1,* Volumes 1 and 2, 2001.

Kumar V, Cotran RS, Robbins SL, Stanley L: *Basic Pathology,* 5th ed. Philadelphia, WB Saunders, 1992.

Levinson WE, Jawetz E: *Medical Microbiology and Immunology.* East Norwalk, CT, Appleton & Lange, 1994.

Moore KL: *Clinically Oriented Anatomy,* 3rd ed. Baltimore, Williams & Wilkins, 1992.

Mycek MJ, Gartner SB, Perper MM: *Pharmacology.* Philadelphia, JB Lippincott, 1992.

Netter FH: *Atlas of Human Anatomy,* 6th ed. West Caldwell, NJ, Ciba-Geigy Medical Education, 1993.

Schneider AS, Szanto PA: *Pathology.* Baltimore, Williams & Wilkins, 1993.

Shayman JA: *Renal Pathophysiology.* Philadelphia, JB Lippincott, 1995.

Weir J, Abrahams PH: *An Imaging Atlas of Human Anatomy.* Aylesbury, Great Britain, Wolfe Publishing, 1992.

Index

Page numbers in *italics* denote figures; those followed by "t" denote tables.